Dying, Yet We Live

Dying, Yet We Live

Our Spiritual Care
of the Dying

Paul Chidwick

Anglican Book Centre
Toronto, Canada

1988
Anglican Book Centre
600 Jarvis Street
Toronto, Ontario
Canada M4Y 2J6

Typesetting by Jay Tee Graphics Ltd.

Canadian Cataloguing in Publication Data

Chidwick, Paul
  Dying, yet we live

Bibliography: p.
ISBN 0-919891-91-8

1. Terminal care - Religious aspects -
Christianity. 2. Death. I. Title.

R726.8.C48 1988   261.8'32175   C88-094590-7

Contents

Preface

The purpose of this preface is to introduce myself and my work, so that the reader may know my motivation for writing this book, what methods and materials were used to procure the information, and whom it was written for. The last is most important since one could easily assume that it is only for professional pastoral caregivers. This is not the case. For reasons which will become evident in the succeeding chapters, the book is designed for anyone who may be called upon to offer care to the terminally ill.

The book was conceived out of a sense of frustration. During my twenty-eight years as a parish priest and teacher in pastoral theology, and the last ten years working with the terminally ill through the parish of St. Mary's and the Hospice of Windsor, I discovered that there was a great deal of misunderstanding about what spirituality involved and who might be called upon to offer spiritual care. The parameters of spiritual care were often limited to things ecclesiastical and circumscribed within the role description of a particular professional group. The main thesis of this book is that our concept of spirituality needs to be broadened, and that this will greatly affect the identity of the caregivers.

There is a bias in the way the data was gathered. I made every attempt to gather as much material as possible from Canadian sources. Admittedly the literature on the subject was scarce, but there was much to be learned from individuals and groups who were already providing care in this field. Their contribution towards the contents of this book needs to be acknowledged. I wish to thank the chaplains and staff of the palliative care programme at St. Clare Mercy Hospital and the Janeway Hospital, St. John's, Newfoundland; the chaplains and co-ordinators of Hospice Services and Pastoral Care at Victoria General Hospital and the Halifax Infirmary, Halifax, Nova Scotia; Dr. Nancy Grant at the Hospice of St. John, St. John, New Brunswick; Dr. Phyllis Smyth, Chaplain at the Royal Victoria Hospital, Montreal; Dr. John Scott, Women's College Hospital, Toronto; Dr. Margaret Scott, Grace Hospital, Toronto; Dr. Dorothy Ley and the staff of the Palliative Care Foundation, Toronto; Wilma O'Connell and the pastoral caregivers at St. Vincent de Paul Hospital, Brockville, Ontario; Dr. Paul Henteleff, St. Boniface Hospital, Winnipeg, Manitoba; Dr. William Lamers, formerly Tom Baker Cancer Centre, Calgary, Alberta, together with the chaplains of the Calgary area; Dr. Helen Hayes, Edmonton General Hospital, Edmonton, Alberta; and Ruthella Graham, Hospice Victoria, Royal Jubilee Hospital, Victoria, British Columbia.

I am particularly grateful for the editorial work of Dr. Balfour Mount, Dr. Dorothy Ley, and Dr. Cope Schwenger. Their frank and incisive comments greatly improved the final draft of the manuscript. I am indebted to the people of St. Mary's Church, Windsor, for allowing me to take a sabbatical and begin writing, and also to one particular individual whose assistance made the sabbatical possible. The experience of working with the terminally ill at the Hospice of Windsor over the past six years helped me immensely in the preparation of this book.

The title *Dying Yet We Live* is a paraphrase from the writings of St. Paul (2 Corinthians 6:9). In this passage St. Paul speaks about how he and his followers have suffered many tribulations but have faced them with "steadfast endurance," a phrase which really does not do justice to the original language. The word *endurance* here does not imply a kind of passive resignation whereby people stoically allow the troubles of life continually to buffet them. Instead it suggests facing trials in such a way that a curse becomes a blessing and a tragedy a triumph. Such an attitude can transform life's ignominies into something positive and good. St. Paul could face the constant threat of dying with a spiritual resource that transformed every situation and enabled him to lead a full and meaningful life. It is my belief that, if we are able to tap the spiritual resources of those who are dying, we will enable them to attain a high quality of life for the time that remains — hence, *Dying Yet We Live*.

One further comment regarding the purpose of this book. It is not just for professional pastoral caregivers. It is designed to help all people examine more carefully their concept of spirituality, and to recognize more clearly what part they may play in meeting this particular need of the terminally ill and their families. Anyone could be called upon to be a spiritual confidant. The question is, How well are people prepared to respond to this call? This book is one small contribution towards this preparation.

Introduction

Before I began to write this book I took the opportunity to discuss the subject with some of the leading caregivers in the field. The first thing I noticed was their encouraging and enthusiastic response. There was no hesitation in their minds that matters relating to spirituality and the care of the terminally ill were of paramount importance. I then began to realize that many of the innovators of hospices or palliative care programmes had very deep religious convictions. Most of them had taken time to pursue theological studies and in some cases had also prepared themselves for the ordained ministry. It seemed to me that such a close connection between spirituality and the care of the dying could not be simply a matter of coincidence. I had to investigate further.

While I recognize the fact that there are people engaged in this work who do so out of a sense of social consciousness and have a strong moral desire to provide more care for an often neglected segment of our society, I question whether a person can maintain this work without coming to grips with the deeper spiritual aspects of life. The results of a survey of the Palliative Care Unit at the Royal Victoria Hospital in Montreal tend to confirm this view. This survey attempted to assess the stress factor involved in palliative care work. Dr. David Shepherd briefly summarized the findings in this way.

> Among staff members who did not resign two factors seemed important: the meaning of religion to them (no one who stated that religion was very important resigned) and a venturesome and spontaneous personality. These factors are compatible with the nature of palliative care work which is unique and innovative and calls for an unusual degree of dedication and commitment demanding thereby acceptance of personal risk in giving oneself to others.
> *Canadian Medical Association Journal* 116 (March 1977), p.526

This type of work seems to require people who have acquired a set of religious beliefs or a value system which is integrated and influential in their lives.

I wanted to discover why the innovative leaders in palliative care thought their spiritual life was so fundamental to the work they were doing. I wrote to them; and again, to my surprise and delight, everyone responded.

There were certain common themes running through their replies which I would like to share with you (I do not place them in any order of priority). The first was the recognition that palliative care demands a holistic approach. Dr. Derek Doyle of St. Columba's Hospice in Edinburgh comments: "I doubt whether a person can practice holistic care without a profound awareness of the spiritual dimension of life and the spiritual needs of fellow men and women." This was echoed by Dr. David Skelton, who was responsible for establishing the Palliative Care Unit at St. Boniface Hospital in Winnipeg. He believes that, on the whole, the people engaged in this work are "deeply caring individuals interested in holisitic approaches to health care." In a very personal comment, Dr. John Scott at Women's College Hospital, Toronto, spoke of his concern to combine his spirituality with this work. He said: "I had a desire to integrate Christian concepts of wholeness into the way I practice medicine. Hospice allows me to integrate my life, i.e. my dual professional training and my personal struggle to integrate faith and work."

Another common theme centred around the concept of service. Dr. Balfour Mount of the Royal Victoria Hospital in Montreal comments: "I don't think it would be possible for a person to do this work unless they had a high need to serve." And he goes on to say that it is within the acts of serving that a person meets the spiritual dimensions of life. "To care for the terminally ill is, for the Christian, to find him (Christ) standing by your side as a member of the team, lying in the bed in the heart of suffering, and standing by the bedside as a loved one engulfed in grief."

Dr. Derek Doyle adds another dimension to this high need to serve and suggests another motivating factor in the spiritually minded person. "Religious people, of any faith, have a deep, innate sense of sacrifice in the service of others, almost a martyr syndrome, and thrive on doing what others will not dare to do, and suffering, not always in silence, is part of the price for this dedicated service. Many of the leaders of the hospice movement that I have met undoubtedly share some evidence of a martyr syndrome." In many ways I would agree with this observation. It reflects the thoroughly engrained work ethic of many people who believe that, unless there is an element of struggle and hardship in service to others, God will not be particularly pleased.

An interesting observation was made by Dr. John Scott as he tried to compare his approach to that of a humanist. He said: "While some humanists are certainly part of the movement, the failure of humanistic philosophy to adequately deal with death is a great deterrent. The relative lack of fear of personal death in the Christian frees him to work with the dying with less anxiety." This was a thought shared by Dr. Doyle. "People with a deep religious conviction, of whatever faith, have a sense of the non-finality of death, knowing that life follows death which, therefore, to some extent, loses its sting. I believe that many Christians are more comfortable than non-believers would be in the presence of death."

Probably the most widely shared comments focused on the search for meaning. Respondents felt that the circumstances surrounding the life of a dying person provide for a natural encounter with what is truly meaningful in life, and they identified this as the connecting factor between spirituality and their work. Dame Cicely Saunders of St. Christopher's Hospice in England writes: "My main answer to the connection between spirituality and palliative care would be a perpetual search for meaning which in the Christian field means a discovery of the compassionate vulnerability of God." Her colleague at St. Christopher's, Dr. Tom West, shares the same concern: "Unless we can see some meaning behind and beyond this life, it will be hard for us not to go stale, become superficial, or burn out. The alternative to seeing some meaning is to continue to search for some meaning. Thinking of myself and those that I work with, it is possibly even more important that we continue to search than assume either that there is any meaning or that we have arrived."

Dr. Skelton explains how this search for meaning is drawn out of the caregivers. "With the passage of time, close proximity to the patients facing severe losses engenders discomfort within the caregivers and causes them to examine very broad issues such as faith and the centrality of reserves and strengths which transcend the human personality. I feel this leads to a fairly universal law of increased spirituality among the workers." This challenge to face life's realities is expressed by Dr. Mount: ("Standing in the arena of death causes one to reflect on life's four essential existential questions: life's meaning, our frightening freedom, our essential aloneness, and the existence of death.') He continues: "We all have a spiritual dimension to our lives that is brought into sharper focus when the illusions of life are swept away by confrontation with death. As caregivers working in this field, such questions gain greater significance for us as we are challenged to examine their implication in our own lives."

Finally, there was one word continually used to describe innovators in the field of palliative care, the word *missionary*. Sometimes this word can be used in a pejorative sense. Dr. Doyle drew attention to the fact that sometimes people can manifest a "missionary zeal which borders on fanaticism. I therefore suggest that people with such obsessional personalities, sanctioned by their religious convictions, find a ready-made place for them in palliative care." As a former missionary I take this comment as a warning rather than as a criticism. I think I would agree with John Scott that hospice pioneers in each country share a "missionary mentality." He says that he chose this new and adventuresome work for the simple reason that it presented an "exciting new 'mission field' in the midst of North American health care."

I have a high regard for the words *mission* and *missionary* because they convey an image of someone who has not only discovered something good in life but also is willing to share it. I think it is much easier to temper a person's enthusiasm with clear, rational judgement than to instill a sense of dedicated service in someone who may have all the academic understanding of a particular cause but lacks commitment. Any new endeavour will have its share of zealots. But maybe they are hearing the words of Isaiah: "The zeal of the Lord of Hosts shall do this" (Isaiah 9:7). I would consider such "informed" zeal to be an important connecting point between one's spirituality and the care of the dying.

When I reflect on my own attitude towards death and the acceptance of it, I recall certain experiences I have had over the years which have revealed something significant about my own spiritual life. I need to explain this in a somewhat roundabout manner. I am a great lover of music and there are certain passages which

I find exquisitely beautiful. When I hear them I often say to myself: "If I could compose something like that and leave it for posterity, even anonymously, I would die content." I do not really believe that this reaction is the product of my desire to achieve immortality. I rather believe that it is a desire to discover and realize something meaningful in my own life. It is my search for fulfilment in life, a search which I know will never be complete, but will have moments when I can say it has been worthwhile. From the very beginning of my work in palliative care I have had a great concern that those people who are facing the end of their earthly existence have the kind of support which will enable them to search for meaning and purpose in their own lives. I believe that this search is an opportunity to bring one's spirituality into focus.

I must also admit that I share with John Scott a fascination for this new and adventuresome mission field. I recall a statement made by my father which probably reveals something about my own spirituality. Besides being a priest he was also an excellent artist, and when I asked him about how he felt when he sold a painting he replied: "It doesn't bother me to see it go. My excitement does not lie in the finished product — it is in the blank canvas." I share in that kind of creativity which so characterizes the field of palliative care.

If I were to single out one reason for engaging in this work, it would be the personal rewards which I have received from those who were supposedly under my care. I have found myself in the company of people for whom the trivia and superficialities of life are of no consequence. Those things which are truly valuable in life have dominated our thoughts and conversations, with the result that I have had the joy of establishing many loving and trusting relationships. It has been within the context of death that I have learned how to live. It has been no sacrifice for me to minister to the dying. It has become my privilege.

When we reflect on the history of palliative care, we find that it was either the work of one professional group, such as monks and nuns in the medieval church, or a combination of such people within the extended family. Even in our own century it was the doctor who often served as both counsellor and spiritual advisor, besides acting as a medical practitioner. The responsibility for addressing the total needs of a patient often rested with one person. But certain factors have altered the situation radically.

In many instances the extended family is no longer a viable support group. The transient nature of our society has fragmented the family, and the terminally ill are left with a limited number of family members to care for them. Advanced medical knowledge has led to increased specialization, and the majority of terminally ill patients end up in institutions where they receive care from a variety of specialists. We have doctors, pain-control specialists, nurses, social workers, psychologists, and pastoral caregivers, each with their own expertise, trying to meet the total needs of the patient. One of the biggest questions facing us now is how all these disciplines can be interrelated so that the patient is treated not in segments but as a whole person.

And where does spirituality fit into the scheme of things? How does the pastoral caregiver relate to the rest of the team? Is spiritual care a specialty reserved for one professional group, or is it a shared concern? What are the boundaries of pastoral care, and where does it overlap with other disciplines? These and similar questions have prompted caregivers to seek a relevant and meaningful place for spirituality in the care of the dying.

This book is an attempt to address these questions. In chapter 1 we will consider some of the contemporary definitions of spirituality and how they might relate to other disciplines. Chapter 2 will focus on the spiritual issues most often raised by patients and their families. This will lead us in chapter 3 to consider who is responsible for dealing with these spiritual issues. Particular attention will be given to the role of the patient. In chapter 4 we will consider some of the unique spiritual phenomena which some dying patients may experience, and also try to provide some kind of theological reflection on the significance of these experiences. Chapter 5 is more practical in nature and will consider some of the appropriate pastoral responses to a patient's spiritual needs. Finally, a concluding chapter will look at the future of spirituality in the care of the dying.

I hope that this book will stimulate all caregivers, be they professionals, volunteers, or family members, to clarify in their minds what spiritual care really involves, and so enable them to recognize their part in providing this kind of care. I also hope that the issues raised will provoke further discussion and encourage others to provide additional insights on this subject.

What Is Spirituality?

Spirituality does not currently occupy a very respectable place in our health care system. One glaring illustration of this fact is the absence of pastoral-care services in many of our hospitals. Most often the chaplain is the last to be hired and the first to be fired. In a survey of over three hundred hospitals in the United States, reaching nearly a thousand health-care professionals, Joseph Fichter concludes "that the great majority of physicians and surgeons — even in church related hospitals — simply have little or no confidence in the spiritual dimension of sick care."[1]

Such a conclusion is not surprising. Medicine is a practical science and deals with those things which can be measured and quantified. It is very difficult, if not impossible, to apply the same approach to the field of spiritual care. As a result, caregivers in these two professions will tend to measure the value of their work differently. A psychological explanation is often used to counter the claim that spiritual intervention has contributed towards the well-being of a patient, and the credibility of spiritual care is consequently damaged. This is not always the fault of medical professionals. Misunderstanding of the place of spirituality in the health-care system can partly be blamed on the pastoral-care workers themselves. Joseph Fichter comments: "It appears that the physicians do not understand the chaplain's role, and that frequently the chaplains cannot explain it to them because they themselves are often not sure of what they are doing."[2]

Even among those people who undertake a holistic approach to medical care, there seems to be a lack of clarity about what spirituality involves. The advocates of palliative care speak about addressing the total needs of the patient. There are the physical needs — and we have a fairly clear idea about how they can be identified and who should deal with these needs. There are the psychological needs — and we are growing in our understanding of how to cope with such emotional pains as denial, anger, anxiety, depression, bargaining, and loneliness. We can understand the social needs and endeavour to treat patients in such a way that they do not feel totally abandoned by the community. We then look to spiritual needs, and it sometimes seems as if this category has been added to cover anything left over that we had forgotten.

In some cases spiritual care appears to be a very limited and church-related activity. We picture a cleric wearing the appropriate apparel, carrying a Bible or suitable religious literature, saying prayers and dispensing ceremonial rites related to his or her denomination. We expect that, when the cleric moves from urbane pleasantries to a topic of spiritual concern, the conversation will contain statements about one's faith in God, one's belief in the next life, or one's readiness to meet one's maker. This may appear to be a somewhat flippant description of spirituality, and I certainly do not intend to belittle this approach. But it is regrettable that spirituality should be limited to saving a person from the clutches of a judgemental God or to making sure that there are no outstanding debts which would jeopardize the chance of entering heaven.

Certainly a person's salvation is of ultimate importance, but never having witnessed a death-bed conversion, I wonder about the fruitfulness of this approach. There is evidence that personal faith can be strengthened at this time, but very seldom is there a complete change of heart or a reversal of one's personal attitude towards religion. This is not to say that it cannot happen; but to identify spirituality only in terms of conversion is to limit the scope of spiritual care and ignore a person's total spiritual needs. Spirituality is a much broader subject.

Current Definitions of Spirituality

In a recent article Alan Tipping defines spiritual care for the dying: "The word *spiritual* can be something of a block if we do not have a clear understanding of the word. I like to describe *spiritual* as referring to the gift of God's spirit which is given to us. It means our openness to God's spirit, our relationship to God and others, and how we are motivated and sustained by the spirit of God. In short *spiritual* refers to relationships which are horizontal — self and others, and those that are vertical — self and God. The dying person is completing the process that will terminate, not in death, but in completeness that follows death. While many dying people may not consciously appreciate what this means to them, the needs they express draw them forth in the process that leads to wholeness and a completeness of life. The pastor or spiritual caregiver assists the dying in this process."[3]

The crucial word in this description is *relationships*. Most often our discussions of spirituality are couched in religious terminology. But a person can have considerable knowledge about religion without being the least bit spiritual. We need words to communicate with each other, but they have to be expressed in the context of daily living before we can say that we are engaged in some kind of spiritual activity. John Scott has succinctly summarized this idea. "The focus of spirituality is not a philosophy but relationships. Spirituality is involved in our horizontal relationships."[4] "We so often consider spirituality to be ethereal and other-worldly. Yet true spirituality is concerned with love as it is expressed in concrete historical situations."[5]

Many pastoral caregivers define their role in terms of relationships. One of the scriptural texts which they are fond of quoting is 1 John 4:20.

> But if a man says "I love God", while hating his brother, he is a liar. If he does not love the brother whom he has seen, it cannot be that he loves God whom he has not seen.

This text suggests that our love for God acquires visibility in our love for one another. We enter the realm of spirituality within the context of a loving relationship — the arena where the spiritual presence of God can be experienced.

Another broad interpretation of the dimensions of spiritual care has been compiled by the National Hospice Organization of the United States. In their standards of hospice-care programme they define the spiritual component in this way.

> Hospice care is concerned with the dynamic process of religion, that is with binding together, tying up, and tying fast. On the intrapersonal level, Hospice endeavors to support the integration of the human personality in the face of the physical deterioration in impending death. The intrapersonal dimension of hospice care seeks to promote the development and continuance of significant human relationship(s) between the dying person and other human beings. And finally, in regard to the eschatological dimension of human life, hospice care affirms

each person's search for ultimate meaning by respecting and responding to each individual's personal truth.[6]

When a number of hospice caregivers were given the opportunity to explain their role as spiritual counsellors, they listed the following points. "Hospice caregivers think that spiritual care involves respecting the diverse beliefs of patients; being willing to discuss spiritual concerns and to explore questions of meaning; making available the comforts or rituals of conventional religion; supporting patients' efforts to make peace with themselves, others and God; and being on hand and letting patients know that they are loved."[7] It is refreshing to find that, while conventional religious activities are recognized, there is an appropriate concern for such things as establishing relationships and the search for meaning.

Spirituality as Becoming a Human Being

All people have a spiritual life by virtue of their existence as human beings. If we were to define what it means to be a human being, we would, in fact, be describing what it means to be spiritual. This is obviously a very broad statement and needs considerable clarification.

The crucial question that needs to be addressed is, What does it mean to be human? Nietzsche said, "He who has a *why* to live can bear with almost any *how*." This was a statement which greatly influenced Viktor Frankl as he struggled for meaning in the face of horrible indignity in the concentration camps of Europe. The uniqueness of humanity lies in the willingness and ability to search for meaning — to ask the question Why? In seeking a purpose and explanation for existence, a person exercises a human potential which is truly spiritual. Joseph Fichter comments, "The search for meaning is a characteristic quality of human beings; and one is tempted to suggest that the person acts less than human who proclaims the absurdity and meaninglessness of all existence."[8] It might even be said that a person who has not adopted a set of meaningful beliefs or an integrated value system has forfeited a portion of the human inheritance. There is an important reason for saying this.

Humanity prides itself in the ability to make decisions. Human actions are not just the product of instinctive or emotional reflexes.

One can deliberately choose a course of action. And although this freedom can sometimes be a frightening gift, it is, nevertheless, an integral part of the personality. But it is important to note that decision making never takes place in a vacuum. Behind every decision are certain assumptions which influence a person's judgement. All of us have, over the years, acquired beliefs and values which continually determine our choices. They become the content of a personal religious code. They help us to act responsibly or irresponsibly, depending on how well we have integrated our value system. If we have beliefs which conflict with one another, we will find that we do not have the tools for mature and consistent decision making. A most important human activity is to acquire this integration, to have a value system which promotes harmony, meaning, and purpose in our lives. This process of integration is truly an exercise in spirituality.

For some people this may sound like some kind of humanistic philosophy. Not once has God been mentioned in the course of this description of spirituality. But I do not believe that anything I have said so far is inconsistent with my beliefs about God, or how God interacts with people. But this will require further explanation.

In some Christian traditions God may be pictured as the judgemental figure. God is in heaven keeping a close eye on all we do, and is waiting for us to account for our actions. He is the divine magistrate who dispenses blessings and punishments both in this life and the next. Our job in life is to obey his commands and so avoid his wrath. We know that we will make mistakes, with intent or unwittingly. Consequently we are encouraged carefully to examine ourselves so that we can make acts of penitence and receive God's forgiveness. There is much in the Scriptures and in Christian theology to back up this particular view of our relationship with God. Unfortunately, it seriously limits our understanding of God and fails to provide us with a rationale for living the Christian life.

What we sometimes fail to ask is, Why does God want us to behave in certain ways? What is the purpose of endeavouring to please God with good works? Is the creator simply jealous for our obedience or does God have something else in mind?

There are two passage of Scripture which clarify for me the purpose of human behaviour. St. Paul, in his letter to the Ephesians, explains that God bestows grace on us so that we may '' all at last attain to the unity inherent in our faith and our knowledge of the Son of God — to mature manhood, measured by nothing less than the full stature of Christ'' (4:13). The key phrase is "mature manhood," or in contemporary terms, "mature personhood"; God's ultimate desire for us is that we be fully human. Whatever inspiration God has given over the years in order to help us live a morally responsible life has been designed for our own good. In the Gospel of John, Jesus says, ("I have come that men may have life, and may have it in all its fullness" (John 10:10). For us to realize our true potential, to discover what is good and beautiful within life, to grow into mature personhood, is the rationale for human existence and the purpose God has for us.)

There is an interesting story Christ told his disciples, and it is particularly relevant to our discussion. He spoke of an unclean spirit which came out of a man and, when it could not find another resting place, decided to return to its original home. When it got there, it found the home unoccupied and swept clean. As a result it went and found seven other spirits worse than itself, and they all entered and dwelt there. And the last state of that man was worse than the first.

It is a strange story; the man would have been better off if he hadn't got rid of the evil spirit in the first place. Perhaps we could conclude that it is not sufficient for us to root out our inadequacies and those things which prevent us from mature personhood, unless we plant something else in their place. The Christian faith has so often been presented as a religion of cleansing, rejecting the negative aspects of life; too little attention has been paid to the positive and upbuilding qualities which enable us to develop human personality and find meaning in life. Consequently, to look for what is good, upbuilding, and meaningful in our life is not a matter of pride or selfishness, but rather an attempt to recognize our spiritual growth and the kind of person we have been and can be. What has this to do with the spiritual care of the dying?

The Search for Meaning and the Life Review

Self-evaluation is a common activity among those who are terminally ill. It is easy to understand why. For the greater part of life we are able to project ourselves into the future. We have dreams and ambitions which provide growth, meaning, and purpose, involving our work, our families, or our efforts to improve our skills and intellectual capabilities. The fact of approaching death does not put an end to this activity completely, but it severely limits a concern for future growth. As Christine Allen has said, ''The structure of meaning that had given shape to our instinct for bearing fruit gets dashed against the wall of death.''[9] This can, of course, lead to serious depression and the belief that life is now meaningless. The dying person desperately needs some kind of spiritual intervention which will help overcome this feeling of meaninglessness.

The problem, and our approach to the problem, has been admirably stated by the same writer.

> The problem for us becomes how to find a new meaning in the days that remain. It is in this context that the instinct to be fruitful and multiply must be turned away from its normal orientation forwards to the future. Instead, it should be focused on a movement *inwards*. In this way, its structure can become infused with a desire for *quality* and *depth* of understanding. This new orientation towards meaning aims to bring about a *re-organization* within the person of information already present. Ultimately it seeks to build an *ordered hierarchy* of values which all relate to each other in some pattern that is satisfying. This satisfaction can lead to a new peace, born and nourished by living fully in the present moment.[10]

This inward movement is sometimes referred to as a life review. Very often it takes the form of personal reminiscences which, in the initial stages, may simply deal with happy events or pleasant acquaintances. But if these reminiscences gain in intensity, they can lead to a complete life review and so make the process of dying meaningful.[11] It has also been discovered that, even though a person may reminisce privately, there is more chance of a satisfactory completion when it is done socially.[12] Herein lies the opportunity for spiritual intervention. The manner in which it is carried out is important. So often death is a managed process in which patients virtually lose control of their dying. By assisting people to complete their life review, we are making some attempt to help them regain more control of their remaining life.

We are inclined to regard the past as something which is gone forever. This is disputable. There is a sense in which the past can never disappear. What we have experienced no power on earth can take away from us. It is our personal heritage which continues to live on in the present. In the words of Viktor Frankl: "Not only our experiences, but all we have done, whatever great thoughts we may have had, and all we have suffered, all this is not lost, though it is past; we have brought it into being. Having been is also a kind of being, and perhaps the surest kind."[13] When people have healthy respect for the past they are able to search for integration and completeness.

It has been discovered that to find integration and meaning in one's life can lead to a sense of peace and harmony, regardless of one's religious belief. Whatever a person's background may be, the search for meaning can become a deeply spiritual activity. Helping people to achieve integration will save them a great deal of spiritual pain. Cicely Saunders has recently said,

> A feeling of meaninglessness, that neither oneself nor the universe has permanence or purpose, is a form of spiritual pain. Patients need to look back over the story of their lives and believe that there was some sense in them and also to reach out towards something greater than themselves, a truth to which they can be committed.[14]

She goes on to say,

> We cannot change what has happened or what we have done but we can come to believe that the meaning of the past can be changed. From this comes the ability to forgive ourselves. This may never be expressed in words on either side but the quality of the ensuing peace is unmistakable.[15]

From an extensive career of working with terminally ill patients, Anne Munley gives practical expression of what actually happens. She says,

> Hospice patients give various indications of movement towards synthesis in the face of impending death. Consistent parts to

this process are efforts mentally to relive life, to assess successes and failures, and to assign meaning to the entire experience.

While visiting patients I spent hours listening to life reviews, I heard warm and bitter memories of childhood, histories of successful and unsuccessful marriages, and tales of offspring which were sources of either pride or shame. I listened to recollections of the work place and of historic events, and to positive and negative memories of encounters with representatives of organized religions. I heard about prosperous times and about times of financial hardship. I listened, too, to accounts of accomplishments, to expressions of regret, to unfulfilled wishes, to admissions of human weakness and failure. Awareness of the present as it was being experienced and subtle reference to the reality of imminent death were always part of these periods of looking back.[16]

It has been recognized that as a person proceeds through this process of looking back and integrating the events of one's life, there can be a growing sense of peace. But the word *peace* can be misleading. In our language the word frequently connotes a calm, tranquil state of mind where everything has come to rest. There is a sense of finality and inactivity. A far better word to describe the integration experience is the Hebrew word *shalom*. It bears connotation of things working together in harmony with each other. It is a dynamic, living word which speaks about a quality of living rather than coming to an end. And surely this is the whole purpose of palliative care — to provide a higher degree of quality in a person's life. To work towards this end is an exercise in spirituality.

It is not unusual for people to speak about finding meaning in life. We reflect on the past and ask, what was the purpose of a particular event? Because we tend to look at life in terms of cause and effect, such questioning is normal. We look back to the source of an event in order to discover its significance and meaning. But there is another way of approaching the issue, and this is important because there can be occasions when it is virtually impossible to see any meaning or purpose. When this happens people can become quite desperate.

It is often possible to add meaning to an event, to put worth or value into an experience, to ascribe purpose rather than to discover it. This is particularly relevant when we are confronted with some inexplicable tragedy. All too often we seem obliged to come up with a reason for everything, and this can result in either a series of pious platitudes (which usually puts the onus on God) or some concocted rationale which leaves the victim of tragedy in a confused and depressed state. If no reason can be determined for the event, then we can simply acknowledge the fact and try to help the person apply some meaning to it.

We all know of situations where the agonizing word *why?* provides little consolation. Tom Harpur, in his book *Harpur's Heaven and Hell*, described a situation where a family had lost its three-month-old child in a crib death. It was an inexplicable tragedy. As the mother said, "He was a perfectly normal baby; there was no warning ahead of time; and no explanation afterwards . . . ." But she went on to say, "I have some comfort in that I know that between Ken and our doctor everything was done that could have been done. What's more, Jason's eyes were given to the eye bank and so, for me, it gives some meaning to his little life." Harpur goes on to comment that "the thought of Jason passing on this gift of sight to someone else has now become for her and Ken the key to turning devastation into hope."[17] This family gave some significance to an otherwise destructive experience.

This could very well be the point Jesus was trying to make when his disciples asked him the question about the blind man: "Rabbi, who sinned, this man or his parents? Why was he born blind?" (John 9:2). The disciples were looking for an explanation to this tragedy. Jesus replied that it had nothing to do with the man himself or his parents but rather "that God's power might be displayed in curing him" (v.3). Jesus put purpose into an inexplicable event.

Finding Meaning in Responsibilities

As we help people search for meaning we may be inclined to focus only on the past and overlook the present and the future, even though the time frame may be limited. Just as some people believe that nothing more can be done for the terminally ill, the terminally ill may also believe that they have nothing to offer anyone else. In actual fact there is much that such a person can do and say — and more will be said about this in a later chapter. The point in raising the issue now is simply to emphasize the need to help a patient recognize and fulfil any responsibilities which he or she may have at the present moment. We must guard against being too over-protective.

Here is a common example of overprotectiveness. Family members are gathered around the patient's bed, and the course of conversation discloses a problem at home or the unexpected arrival of a guest who needs to be housed. At this point the patient begins to offer a solution, but there is the inevitable response: "Oh! Don't worry. We will take care of everything." People say this because they do not want to place any unnecessary burden on the person they love. Undoubtedly they are speaking out of kindness. But there is another message in this response. It says to the patient, "You are all finished with decision making. We have taken over full responsibility. You don't have to think or do anything anymore — just lie there like a vegetable." This is a most regrettable and inhuman message. If it is at all possible, the patient needs to continue being involved in the mainstream of life, which invariably includes making decisions and behaving in a responsible manner.

When we help and allow people to act responsibly, we are giving them the opportunity to exercise their spirituality. We are addressing that part of their human nature which makes them unique — the ability to exercise free will and moral independence. By failing to motivate this spiritual activity we are actually treating them as irresponsible and worthless human beings. We are, in effect, robbing them of their humanity.

The Art of Discovering Meaning

So far we have considered the significance of spirituality from the perspective of the patient. It has been argued that caregivers should make every effort to help the patient engage in his or her search for meaning. But how is this to be done? And who will do it? Some people might say that it is the chaplain's job, since he or she is the supposed expert in the field. But this is not what happens. The fact is that the patient chooses his or her own spiritual counsellor. It could be a nurse, a doctor, a friend, someone from the housekeeping department, another patient — anyone whom the patient feels he or she can trust. This means that all of us have to be prepared to accept the position of a spiritual confidant.

There are certain caregivers who appear to assume this role more than anyone else. They are primarily the nurses, the orderlies, and the domestic staff of the hospital. Derek Doyle of St. Columba's Hospice in Edinburgh agrees, "It is medical and nursing staff who first encounter problems which may broadly be defined as spiritual."[18] Even though there are three experienced chaplains at St. Columba's Hospice, Dr. Doyle estimates that about 80 per cent of their patients chose someone other than the chaplain to discuss spiritual matters. This may have something to say about the role of the chaplain or the image people have of the chaplain (which I shall discuss later), but one of the primary reasons is accessibility. Since spiritual issues do not emerge at any specified time, it is the most accessible person who will be called upon to assume the role of a spiritual confidant.[19] Some people may feel uncomfortable assuming this role, and so it is important that we consider appropriate ways of meeting people on this level.

Christine Allen outlines the process whereby two people bridge the gulf and so establish a relationship which enables both persons to pursue their search for meaning.

> In the first place we are faced with two people, separate and distinct, with a combined framework of meaning and energy. The gulf of meaning gaps wide between them.

> Next an attempt is made at building a common ground. The foundation for the bridge across the gulf is laid.

> Then differences begin to be explored. The bridge becomes built so that passage is able to occur in both directions.

> Either or both persons may be affected by a growth of level of integration and by the discovery of a renewed meaning structure which is satisfying and brings a certain inner peace. There is a constant possibility of travel back and forth. The gulf of meaning no longer seems important.

> Finally, in certain situations something new is created by the relationship, something which goes beyond the original two

people involved. At this moment not only has the bridge over the gulf of meaning been built, and used, but a union of the two extremities of the bridge has brought forth a new entity. The bridge has assumed a life of its own.

This new life, when it occurs, is experienced as coming from outside, as a kind of grace. It cannot be predicted or controlled. In a sense it cannot even be worked for, as its presence is unexpected and known only "after the fact." We must not expect that the bridges we try to build will always or even often come alive. It is important to keep reminding ourselves in this particular work with serious illness and death that we are only able to lay the foundation for bridges. In so far as we take responsibility for the quality of our own lives we will bring to the bridge-making a certain possibility of result. The ultimate nature of the bridge itself, however, will be determined by the mysterious interaction of the other persons involved. There is always a factor of spontaneity present in human life which can overturn all expectation. If we are open to this spontaneity as well as . . . prepared to listen and to give, then there is a chance that something important will occur in the mutual struggle to find meaning in our complex and compelling world.[20]

One very important point which Christine Allen has mentioned is that spiritual counsellors engaged in this search for meaning must have their own house in some reasonable order. The degree to which this has been attained will vary from one person to another. And it may even happen that the patient finds greater integration than the counsellor. The important thing is that the counsellor has endeavoured to achieve some kind of integration in the past and considers the search for meaning to be a relevant activity.

We should not be overcome by the prospect of entering the arena of spiritual care. We can provide spiritual support simply by our love and our actions. Since we are capable of loving and caring, we fulfil the basic criteria for engaging in spiritual growth. We must always remember that spirituality is not confined to words alone. A compassionate presence can also provide spiritual support. Viktor Frankl expresses it in this way:

Love is the only way to grasp another human being in the innermost core of his personality. No one can become fully aware of the very essence of another human being unless he loves him. By the spiritual act of love he is enabled to see the essential traits and features in the beloved person; and even more, he sees that which is potential in him, that which is not yet actualized but yet ought to be actualized. Furthermore, by his love, the loving person enables the beloved person to actualize these potentialities. By making him aware of what he can be and of what he should become, he makes these potentialities come true.[21]

Consequences of the Search for Meaning

We might ask at this point about the kind of spiritual growth we might expect to see in a patient as he or she engages in the search for integration and meaning. There has been a lot of interest in trying to discover whether the religious life of people enables them to cope with impending death, and whether there are any dramatic changes to be expected at this time. It seems to be generally agreed that there are few death-bed conversions, a conclusion which I have also reached after many conversations with pastoral caregivers.[22] Some people have said that the religious life which people bring into the hospital is what they leave with. This is possibly an oversimplified remark, but it indicates that people do not try to play games with God at this point in their life. What can happen is an intensification of faith and an openness to discuss the religious values which have been acquired over the years. This is not to infer that there will be no growth at all, it is simply that matters relating to the religious life are taken more seriously and articulated more freely. John Hinton has shown in his book *Dying* that people with strong faith and people with no faith exhibited less anxiety about death than people with tepid faith.[23] Those who have made efforts to integrate their religious beliefs, and who have built a sound value system during their days of living, appear better able to cope than those who leave it until their days of dying.

It may seem strange to some people that my overall remarks about spirituality contain only passing mention to specific religious beliefs and practices. This has been done deliberately if only to suggest to readers that they have probably, on many occasions, been engaged in conversations relating to spirituality but would not have identified them as such at the time. So often specific denominational beliefs do not allow us to examine the subject from a total perspective. In my experience, patients and their families show little or no interest in those issues which characterize a particular denomination. It is not that they consider them worthless, but they feel the need to go beyond these issues to something far more basic, issues which are not contained in catechisms or particular rites and practices. For this reason I have assumed a very broad definition of spirituality. The truth about God and man can never be fully expressed in any one religious system. We are dealing with a great mystery, and it would seem that the people about to leave this world find themselves very close to becoming a part of that mystery. It is within this context that my understanding of spirituality has been developed.

Spirituality and Psychotherapy

It is quite possible, however, that a broad-based definition of spirituality could lead to some confusion. Many helpful spiritual interventions are sometimes labelled as good psychotherapy. It is important, therefore, to explore the difference between spiritual and psychological care.

It would be far too simplistic to say that the psychologist is concerned only with the measurable causative factors of particular emotional states, while the pastoral caregiver is primarily concerned about values, meaning, and the purpose of life. Many of the issues raised by patients today, which in former years would normally have been referred to a priest, are now being directed towards other medical personnel. This can make them feel uncomfortable, especially if they view their profession in purely technical terms. They may resist any involvement in areas which call for some philosophical or religious response. While I may have a certain sympathy with medical personnel, at the same time I think that they are abdicating an important responsibility. It is certainly true that a doctor can simply treat the biological mechanism without relinquishing his or her status as a doctor, but I believe that the medical practitioner should be prepared to take seriously other factors in the patient's condition, even though these may include the spiritual. This is the only way that complete and proper care can be achieved. Of what profit is it if a surgeon amputates a leg only to find that the patient commits suicide because he or she cannot accept the disfigurement or the loss of function. Surely there is a place for the patient to be assured that he or she can still live a valuable and meaningful life in spite of this disability.

But the question remains, When should the doctor address the spiritual needs of the patient and When should this be left to the spiritual director? Or can the doctors divorce themselves completely from certain spiritual responsibilities? Hippocrates once said, "One must bring philosophy to medicine and medicine to philosophy." But doesn't this imply that doctors are to bring something foreign into their practice? Are they not exceeding their authority if they engage in some kind of spiritual intervention? And if this is so, where do we draw the line between medical and spiritual care?

I would suggest that part of our problem in answering this question lies in insisting there *should be a line*! It is becoming more apparent every day that the deepest philosophical questions are being asked by scientists as well as theologians. It is commonplace for the student of geophysics to start asking questions about the whys and wherefores of the universe. Today it seems retrogressive to draw too fine a line to mark where one discipline begins and the other ends. There will inevitably be some overlapping. There is a kind of no-man's-land where certain disciplines stand between the frontiers of two countries. But this is not a bad place to be. As long as we are conscious of the limits and parameters of our involvement in a foreign field, we can resist the temptation to enter a sphere where angels fear to tread.

Nevertheless, while recognizing the fact that both psychology and spirituality may overlap at certain points, we still have to face the question regarding their differentiation. The question might be posed in this way. On what grounds would a person consult a psychologist as opposed to a priest? What would be the expectations from each profession in terms of its special expertise? If the question cannot be answered, even with a modest degree of clarity, then it becomes difficult for priest and psychologist to understand their roles in the interdisciplinary care of the patient.

A psychologist would first want to provide a diagnosis of the situation. There would be an attempt to explain why the circumstances arose, identify and evaluate what is presently being experienced, and indicate what may lie ahead in the future if the circumstances persist. At this point the psychologist is providing a data report on the past, present, and future mental condition of the patient. It could stop right there. But the psychologist might also wish to encourage the patient to make some responsible decision that would bring about mental health. This is when the psychologist begins to enter the realm of spirituality, certainly in terms of how it has been described in this chapter. To encourage people to engage in responsible decision making is also asking them to call upon a belief and value system which assists them to make the appropriate decisions. This is an activity in spirituality.

But the next question is, To whom or to what is the patient responsible? To God, to herself, to her conscience, to the community? These are questions of a moral nature, and this is where the spiritual director can help a person find the direction which is consistent with his or her belief and value system. A spiritual director can offer concrete directives as to how the person might act responsibly. They might not be accepted verbatim, but they could provide a basis for decision making.

The psychologist is not expected to prescribe an ethical directive (unless he or she wishes to share a personal belief and value system, but this would indicate that the psychologist has also taken on the role of spiritual director). Responsibility is an ethically neutral concept. One can encourage someone to act responsibly without indicating to what or to whom that person should be responsible. The psychologist may approach spiritual territory by encouraging someone to act in a responsible manner. The spiritual director, on the other hand, can and should point in particular directions as to the way a person could exercise his or her spiritual responsibilities.

In a very clipped statement, Viktor Frankl differentiates the two disciplines in this way. He says, ''The goal of psychotherapy is to heal the soul, to make it healthy; the aim of religion is something essentially different — to save the soul.''[24] It may very well be that to save the soul is to find those behavioural directives which can effect responsible and appropriate decision making. Frankl then goes on to describe his method of psychotherapy which he says borders on the spiritual only in the sense that it prepares a person to act responsibly. He describes what he calls medical ministry in this manner:

> Medical ministry is not ultimately concerned with the "soul's salvation". This could not and should not be its business. Rather, it is concerned with the health of man's soul. And man's soul is healthy so long as he remains what he intrinsically is: namely, a being conscious of his responsibility — in fact, the very vessel of consciousness and responsiblity.[25]

In the introduction to this chapter I quoted Dr. John Scott. It was his desire to "integrate Christian concepts of wholeness into the way I practice medicine." He believes palliative care has allowed him to integrate his life — "my dual professional training and my personal struggle to integrate faith and work." I have attempted to explore this integration, to find a definition of spirituality which is not only consistent with one's beliefs about God and God's purposes for mankind, but can be integrated into the interdisciplinary care of the patient. It has been suggested that the search for meaning, through the encouragement of responsible decisions and actions, can be one spiritual activity which promotes wholeness and quality of life for terminally ill patients and their families. It hardly needs to be said that the place of spirituality in medical care will continue to need more and more clarification. Further attempts will be made when we consider the role of the pastoral caregiver. But first we must examine some of the spiritual issues which are so frequently raised by terminally ill patients.

Notes

1 Joseph H. Fichter, *Religion and Pain* (New York: Crossroad, 1981), p. 123.
2 *Ibid.*, p. 116.

3 Alan Tipping, "Spiritual Care for the Dying," *Canadian Pharmacological Journal* 114 (1981), p. 258.

4 John Scott, "Spiritual Concern," Paper delivered at the Second International Seminar on Terminal Care (Montreal: November 1978), p. 4.

5 *Ibid.*, p. 9.

6 *Standards of a Hospice Program of Care*, National Hospice Organization (McLean, Virginia: 1982), p. 5.

7 Anne Munley, *The Hospice Alternative* (New York: Basic Books, 1983), p. 254.

8 Joseph H. Fichter, *Religion and Pain*, p. 44.

9 Christine Allen, "Bridging the Gap of Meaning: A Philosophical Approach to Palliative Care," *The Royal Victoria Hospital Manual on Palliative/Hospice Care* (New York: Arno Press, 1980), p. 118.

10 *Ibid.*, p. 232.

11 Victor W. Marshall, *Last Chapters, A Sociology of Aging and Dying* (California: Brooks/Cole Publishing Company, 1980), p. 118.

12 *Ibid.*, p. 118.

13 Viktor Frankl, *Man's Search for Meaning* (New York: Pocket Books, 1963), p. 131.

14 Dame Cicely Saunders and Mary Baines, *Living with Dying, The Management of Terminal Disease* (Oxford: Oxford University Press, 1983), p. 63.

15 *Ibid.*, p. 63.

16 Anne Munley, *The Hospice Alternative*, p. 172.

17 Tom Harpur, *Harpur's Heaven and Hell* (Toronto: Oxford University Press, 1983), p. 223.

18 Derek Doyle, ed., *Palliative Care: The Management of Far-Advanced Illness* (London: Groom Helm, 1984), p. 416.

19 Alene Ruth Dickinson, "Nurses' Perceptions of Their Care of Patients Dying with Cancer," Unpublished Ed. D. Dissertation, (Teachers' College, Columbia University, 1966).

20 Christine Allen, "Bridging the Gulf of Meaning: A Philosophical Approach to Palliative Care," p. 240–241.

21 Viktor Frankl, *Man's Search for Meaning*, p. 176.

22 Anne Munley, *The Hospice Alternative*, p. 234.

23 John Hinton, *Dying* (Middlesex, England: Penguin Books, 1967).

24 Viktor Frankl, *The Doctor and the Soul* (New York: Vintage Books, 1973), p. xv.

25 *Ibid.*, p. 277.

Spiritual Issues

People need to find meaning in life. Meaninglessness is, indeed, the greatest spiritual pain. When a person is about to reach the end of his or her life, there will be an even greater need to evaluate the past to discover what has been valuable, what has been accomplished, what contributions have been made to society or individuals. It is during this process of reflection that a person may attain a degree of peace and acceptance. Serious questions are raised at this time, questions which need to be addressed. And even if satisfactory answers cannot be found immediately, the patient needs to have the opportunity to ask. To circumvent this process could present a roadblock towards integration and acceptance of one's condition. To wrestle honestly with these questions could be a turning point in the search for meaning. The question which is probably most frequestly asked, or at least thought about is, What have I done to deserve this? Why me? Whenever this question is raised, either by a patient or a member of the family, it very important to discover whether the person is wanting a theological response to the way God deals with people, or is simply expressing anger at the seeming injustice of the situation. Very often these questions are simply a verbal outburst of deep emotional feeling. It is crucial that this be determined before one engages in a theological dissertation on the doctrine of providence or the righteousness of God. As Susan Quinn has observed: ''Many hospice patients and families, regardless of their religious affiliation, ask spiritual questions . . . . The issues and the feelings that accompany these questions are best handled by the chaplain, but any trained staff member on the team can also help the patient or family member. Listening to the patient explore feelings is usually what is needed. Answers are generally not sought or required.''[1]

Another similar question often heard is, Why is God doing this to me? Or if the question comes from a family member it can take the form, Why does God allow her to suffer so much? And when the end has come, Why did God let him die? These can also be cries of anguish or a search for some meaning and purpose. Our initial response must always be to determine what the person is actually asking.

Besides questions one also hears statements which reflect a patient's attempt to find some kind of resolution to a very difficult situation. We might even call them attempts to explain the mystery of death. "I guess my time is up. I suppose these things are sent to try me. God knows best." These can be expressions of resignation to the inevitable circumstances of life or they can be questions in disguise. The person could be testing out a possible answer and looking for a response. Even the remark, "I guess the next life will be better than this one," may be a profession of faith in the afterlife, or it may be a roundabout way of asking the question, Is there really another life after death?

This is not to imply that every question is suspect or that patients are never really interested in a serious and thoughtful response. The point is simply to warn caregivers to be quite clear as to what the patient is really asking. We must proceed in a very sensitive and loving manner when we respond to these questions.

There are some very disturbing responses which have caused more damage than good. Very well-meaning spiritual counsellors have appealed to Scripture and quoted the words of Job when he was given the news that his entire family had been killed: "The Lord gives and the Lord takes away; blessed be the name of the Lord" (Job 1:21). Some may comment, "God knows when it is time to depart this world." The assumption lying behind these responses is that every person's death has been pre-ordained by God and that the method and timing is entirely in God's hands. This might be a comforting thought for a ninety-five-year-old widow who has lived a full life and has little reason to continue, but it is small consolation for a young couple who have been told that their child has been killed by a drunken driver.

Sometimes a counsellor may say, "God has taken her away" or "God needs her more than you do." Here the listener may infer that the departed is better off dead than alive, which doesn't say anything very complimentary about his or her former relationship with the bereaved. Indeed, such comments could instill feelings of guilt or anger that God had finally rescued that person from a very unhappy environment.

All these statements are attempts to provide comfort for the bereaved and to suggest some kind of rationale for the tragic event. But the theological basis for these remarks, and the fact that God is being represented as some capricious deity arbitrarily giving and taking life when it suits the divine purpose, are open for question. Those who make these remarks are quick to remind us that one day we will understand the reason for these apparent tragedies. But surely we are not asked to believe that God will provide us with a *good* reason why millions of Jews were *taken away* to the gas chambers during the last world war? There are times when our pious platitudes help people endure the pain of separation, but there are also times when they make absolutely no sense at all. And if there is not some consistent truth underlying such statements, a truth which can be applicable to the whole gamut of tragic events, then there is something radically wrong with the underlying theological suppositions.

A very useful comment was made by John Swift in an article on the role of the chaplain. He speaks about healthy and unhealthy beliefs. "A religious belief and practice which enhances life and provides nourishment for growth (even in the process of dying) is a healthy one; one which stifles life and handicaps growth is unhealthy."[2] He goes on to quote Howard J. Clinebell, who suggests the kind of questions one might ask to separate health-producing from health-retarding beliefs and practices. He says, "Does a particular religious belief and practice: build bridges between people rather than barriers? build respect for the emotional and intellectual levels of life? show concern for the health of personality rather than for surface behaviour? provide clear moral and ethical guidelines and provide effective means of handling guilt? emphasize growth and love rather than fear? provide an adequate frame of reference and object of devotion?"[3] These are, I think, the kind of questions which need to be faced if we are to validate an effective and meaningful response. It is sometimes the case that the belief systems underlying many of the responses to questions raised by the dying and their families are, in fact, considerably unhealthy. They arouse suspicions about God, fear of coming into God's presence, guilt about past relationships, and certainly they show little respect for the intellectual level of the persons concerned. We should manifest a great deal more care in determining the theological implications of our responses. Let us take a look at some of the significant beliefs underlying these statements.

The Nature of God

The first and foremost belief we have to consider is about the nature of God. Much of what we have learned goes back to early childhood and was acquired partly through formal religious education but fundamentally through the teaching and example of our parents. Harold Kushner wrote his book *When Bad Things Happen to Good People* in response to the tragic death of his son; he began by reflecting on what he believed was a typical image of God. He said, "Like most people, my wife and I had grown up with an image of God as an all-wise, all-powerful parent figure who would treat us as our earthly parents did, or even better. If we were obedient and deserving, he would reward us. If we got out of line, he would discipline us, reluctantly but firmly. He would protect us from being hurt or from hurting ourselves, and would see to it that we got what we deserved in life."[4] This is a fairly accurate description for the majority of religiously minded people. In so many ways we project on to God those attributes which characterize the authority figures in our lives. Fathers have assumed the role of decision makers, disciplinarians, providers, and the ones who make the final judgements. Fathers are not usually the ones who give comfort in times of sickness, nourishment when you are hungry, or a bosom to cry on when you are hurt or frightened. Consequently, God assumes more of the male characteristics than female, and is pictured primarily as a judgemental figure. As this image has instilled fear in the minds of children, it is not uncommon for adults to manifest a similar fear in their relationship with God.

John Shanahan traces this attitude towards God back to the medieval period when, in both art and literature, Christ is depicted as "the judge of all men at whose feet stands humanity definitively judged — rewarded or condemned — the just called to heaven, the wicked consigned to hell. Because this popular piety of the late medieval period has been so prominent in my religious community until recently, I have seen and shared these same tensions with those who are about to die."[5] This appears to be the experience of most caregivers. The pervading image of God in the minds of many patients is the judgemental figure. The patient may not actually verbalize this in so many words, but it is the underlying assumption in such questions as, What did I do to deserve this? or, Why me? This image also comes to mind very naturally when a person undertakes a life review. The whole process of weighing out checks and balances is an exercise in personal evaluation which is not only a search for meaning, but can also be an act of self-judgement. It is only natural for a person to mirror his or her findings against what God expects. And the judgement of God begins right there! As man seeks for some justification of his life, God comes to mind as the one seeking justice.

The same point is taken by Richard Lamerton. "A man in extremis knows he can't get away with anything, that God is not mocked. If he knows about Justice (as in Britain everyone does) he may reasonably be terrified. And the only consolation he can possibly be given in the light of this knowledge is to be reminded that Justice is only an aspect of mercy, that this is the first quality radiated by the Godhead, and that it is boundless, without measure."[6] As true as these words may be, it is no easy task to alter one's image of God when it has been engraved in a particular fashion since childhood. One would hope that besides words of comfort there would be actions which would reveal the true nature of the Godhead. As one patient remarked about the care he was receiving in the Palliative Care Unit at Grace Hospital in Toronto: "When I entered this place I forgot the God of my childhood and discovered the true nature of God." The righteous, omnipotent, and omniscient God had been found to be also a God of love, compassion, and mercy.

Suffering and the God of Love

But this does raise the age-old question. How can we reconcile the concept of a good and all-powerful God with the experience of unmerited suffering? This question, commonly known as theodicy, has plagued the minds of theologians for centuries. If God is all-powerful, then everything that happens in life is under divine direction. Consequently, when evil things befall us or we contract a life-threatening illness, we have to believe that God is still in control of the situation. And since God is also righteous and would never commit any injustice against humanity, we are forced to ask why God would bring on this misfortune. And so we begin the desperate search for answers.

The tragic event may be explained as a punishment. This is probably the thought behind the question, What have I done to deserve this? People have suggested that God may be testing our faith or teaching us a lesson, and that this is a way of promoting our spiritual growth. Bishop Jeremy Taylor, in his *Rules of Holy Dying*, reflects the belief that there is a direct relationship between the suffering of a sinner and God's therapeutic activity. In his mind there were potential benefits in the agonies of the dying: "Certain it is, that a mourning spirit and an afflicted body are great instruments of reconciling God to a sinner, and they always dwell at the gates of atonement and restitution" (8, p.372). A more recent theologian, the Rev. Joseph Sullivan, contends that the mental agony of approaching death is "part of the sacrifice that God demands for the sins and faults of life . . . some suffering is necessary; God knows how much each man needs."[7] Unfortunately, these explanations do nothing to help us understand why the innocent suffer. The only purpose they serve is to vindicate, at all costs, the justice of God. And this is particularly distressing since so many patients look upon their suffering as a form of punishment. Such statements only enhance their feelings of guilt.

There is an old adage which is reflected in so much of the Old Testament writings that "the wicked suffer and the righteous prosper." And when it was observed that there were innocent people suffering and wicked people doing well in the world, it was simply explained that sooner or later the wicked would suffer, either in this world or the next. The psalmist wrestled with this problem. He says, "My feet had almost slipped, my foothold had all but given way, because the boasts of sinners roused my envy when I saw how they prosper. So wicked men talk, yet still they prosper and rogues amass great wealth" (73:2–3,12). But he consoles himself, "How often thou dost set them on slippery ground and drive them headlong into ruin! Then in a moment how dreadful their end, cut off root and branch by death with all its terrors" (73:18–19). Sooner or later the wicked will get their deserts.

This was the same problem which Job had to face. The scenario at the beginning of the book seems to indicate that the dreadful things which happened to Job were meant to test his faith. Job himself cannot fathom what heinous crimes he could have committed to warrant such suffering. His three friends, with their somewhat shallow sophistry, continue to argue that he must have sinned because God is righteous and just. For thirty-eight chapters Job bemoans his fate. And then comes God's reply.

> Where were you [Job] when I laid the earth's foundations?
> Tell me, if you know and understand.
> Who settled its dimensions? Surely you should know. (38:4-5)
> Can you bind the cluster of the Pleiades
> or loose Orion's belt?
> Can you bring out the signs of the zodiac in their season
> or guide Aldebaran and its train?
> Did you procalim the rules that govern the heavens,
> or determine the laws of nature on earth?'' (38:31-33)

There is abundant evidence here that God is asserting his omnipotence over the affairs of the world and is certainly suggesting to Job that there are many mysteries which defy explanation by mortal minds. In the end Job does submit to the unfathomable ways of God, and God rewards him for his faithfulness. But there is another aspect of the discussion which deserves some consideration.

Harold Kushner points out a particular passage in God's response to Job, a passage which adds a new slant to the problem. He writes, ''The most important lines in the entire book may be the ones spoken by God in the second half of the speech from the whirlwind, chapter 40, verses 9-14:

> Have you an arm like God?
> Can you thunder with a voice like His?
> *You* tread down the wicked where they stand,
> Bury them in the dust together . . . .
> Then will I acknowledge that your own right hand
> Can give you victory.''

Kushner continues, ''I take these words to mean 'if you think it is so easy to keep the world straight and true, to keep unfair things from happening to people, *you* try it! God wants the righteous to live peaceful, happy lives, but sometimes even He can't bring that about. It is too difficult even for God to keep cruelty

and chaos from claiming innocent victims. But could man,
without God, do it better?' ''[8]

This seems to suggest that, even though God may be omnipotent, God may deliberately withhold omnipotence in order to
preserve the freedom of man, which, for the most part, is the
cause of most suffering and evil in this world. The passage
declares that God is good, even as Job is good, and that God is
not going to put the blame on Job so that evil can be explained.
But for God to intervene in every distressing or evil situation
would be to disregard the laws of nature and the freedom of man.

I do not believe that Kushner considers this to be the final
answer to the problem, but it does make us reflect on what we
understand omnipotence to be. And whatever we think, it will
inevitably be limited by our finite minds. We can never be absolutely sure how the nature of God is related to the affairs of this
world.

It might be worth noting that the question, What did I do to
deserve this? is really not the appropriate question. Sickness and
death do not come because God decides that we deserve it. The
question we need to ask is, Now that it has happened, what do
I do about it and who is there to help me? Instead of trying to
extract some meaning out of an event, we need to try putting
some meaning into it. This is reflected very beautifully in an old
Jewish prayer written by Levi Yitzchak.

> I do not beg You to reveal to me the secret of Your ways —
> I could not bear it. But show me one thing; show it to me more
> clearly and more deeply: show me what this, which is hap-
> pening at this very moment, means to me, what it demands
> of me, what You, Lord of the world, are telling me by way
> of it. Ah, it is not why I suffer, that I wish to know, but only
> whether I suffer for Your sake.[9]

This does raise the question as to whether there can really be
any value in pain and suffering. Among writers who have wrestled with this question from personal experience Viktor Frankl
stands out clearly. His years of living in the concentration camps
of Europe forced him to face this question. He knew within himself, and watching those around him, that if he did not resolve

the problem he would give up on life and retreat into the apathy of the living dead. Few of us will ever have to face such meaningless horror, and yet through this experience Viktor Frankl has written words which have inspired millions of people.

He is fond of quoting the words of Dostoevski: "There is only one thing that I dread: not to be worthy of my sufferings." These words led him to comment on the lives of those suffering with him: "It can be said that they were worthy of their sufferings; the way they bore their suffering was a genuine inner achievement. It is this spiritual freedom — which cannot be taken away — that makes life meaningful and purposeful . . . . If there is a meaning in life at all, then there must be a meaning in suffering. Suffering is an ineradicable part of life, even as fate and death. Without suffering and death human life cannot be complete."[10]

Suffering is an ineradicable part of life, be it physical, mental, or spiritual. No one will be spared his or her measure of hardship. In the course of history those who have suffered the most and borne it well are heralded as martyrs. We would never have known of them had their lives been smooth and easy. It is also true that of all religions Christianity has presented the endurance of suffering as one of its highest virtues. It has even been proclaimed that those who have suffered the most for their faith in this life receive special honours in the next, and it has been the custom to place them in a closer relationship with God. How valid this is could be debated, but it does indicate that the church has placed significant value in the endurance of suffering.

This has been illustrated recently by Mary Craig in her book *Candles in the Dark*. It is about some latter-day Christian martyrs who have been honoured and commemorated by the Pope, and endorsed by the Archbishop of Canterbury and other leading churchmen. The author does not present these people as perfect and serene. She does not gloss over Dietrich Bonhoeffer's earlier Naziism, or Martin Luther's numerous marital infidelities, or Sister Maria Skobtsova's earlier atheism. These modern saints had a dark side to their lives, but because they died for others they proved themselves to be true martyrs and worthy of commemoration. It would seem that sometimes suffering becomes equated with saintliness.

One wonders whether this is simply a matter of wanting the best for those who have experienced the worst. Or are we saying that as a result of such suffering they have attained a spiritual dignity which demands our respect. And if so, what is this spiritual dignity?

Obviously these people did not suffer for the sake of suffering. There is nothing beautiful or good about pain and death. It should be one of our prime efforts in life to remove pain and suffering. The vision of the next life is expressed exactly in these terms. "(God) will wipe away every tear from their eyes; there shall be an end to death, and to mourning and crying and pain; for the old order has passed away!" (Revelation 21:4). Surely we should attempt to realize in this life what has been promised in the next. Nevertheless, suffering is a fact and we have to deal with it.

It would seem that the spiritual dignity of the true martyr is the example of someone who cannot escape suffering, but is willing to endure it for some purpose. Viktor Frankl once had the opportunity to escape from a prison camp. All the arrangements had been made. Only a matter of hours before his departure he visited his patients for the last time. He was gripped by a terrible conflict. Surely he had suffered enough and should take the opportunity to escape. But who would care for the ones left behind. He decided to stay, knowing that there would be more suffering in the future and even possible death. But he also knew that any further suffering would have a purpose, the care of his fellow prisoners. In his own words: "Suffering ceases to be suffering in some way at the moment it finds a meaning, such as the meaning of a sacrifice."[11] Only those who are able to find some transcendental value in suffering can find meaning in the midst of apparent failure.[12]

Carl Jung once said that "no tree can grow to heaven unless its roots reach down to hell."[13] This sounds as if one cannot grow unless there is a degree of suffering in life, and I am sure that Jung did not mean exactly that. But it is our willingness to enter the abysses of hell which enables us to have a taste of heaven. As we strive through hardship in order to achieve some meaningful end, either for ourselves or others, so we grow into that mature personhood which is the purpose of our spiritual journey.

Among those who have watched others suffer the humiliations and deprivations of dying, Cicely Saunders has had time to reflect on her Christian response to suffering. She finds comfort in the fact that suffering can bring a person into closer union with Christ. She says, "Suffering was — and is — the place where Christ is glorified. He is there whether He is recognized or not. The simple truths that He knows so much better than we ever can, that He knew such dependence that even He had to have His own cross carried for Him, seem to have meaning for the most unaccustomed ears and to need little explanation. I believe that this is because such sufferers are in the place of His deepest identification with us all."[14]

In a very real sense the spirit of Christ is brought into a suffering situation not only by reflecting on his identification with the sufferer but also by the compassionate presence of someone who cares. We can never know with any certainty what the dying person is experiencing. To say to someone, "I know how you feel," is really quite absurd. Even if you were dying yourself, it would be impossible to enter into the inner depths of another person's feelings. But it is important that we indicate to that person how much we would like to understand. When Cicely Sauders asked a patient what it was he needed above all else from those who were caring for him, he said, "For someone to look as if they were trying to understand me."[15] The man knew that it would be impossible for another person to fully understand what he was feeling, but it was a great comfort to know that people were trying. Such effort does much to relieve the anxiety that comes from feeling abandoned.

It is sometimes said that there is a pain that ennobles the human personality and a pain that destroys. There are people who have become the victims of intractable pain or have gone into a severe chronic depression. This can result in personality changes which greatly alarm both the patient and the caregivers. This is the suffering which destroys and we cannot believe for one moment that any good can come from it. Such cases are most regrettable, particularly when one considers just how much suffering could be alleviated if we were prepared to spend more time monitoring the patient. It has been proven beyond any doubt that, in those institutions where some kind of palliative care service is being offered, there is a great reduction in the mental and physical pain of the patients. It has also been documented that when the psycho-social needs are met, which would also include the spiritual, physical pain can be reduced.[16] There is far too much destructive suffering among our patients, and we are at fault. It is not necessarily the case that the patient should have more faith or more courage and so move through this experience to achieve a greater meaning. Pain can destroy people. But so very often it is a pain which could be avoided if our health-care services would exercise more responsibility in this area of care.

Pain and Spirituality

It is not within my province to discuss pain control from the medical point of view. It is, however, quite relevant to our subject to see what effect psycho-social and spiritual interventions can have on the reduction of pain.

For many years it has been recognized by pastoral caregivers that a spiritual intervention, either before or after an operation, has had a positive effect on the recovery of the patient. This is not to say that such interventions will guarantee physical recovery. But even when health does not improve, the patient appears more able to cope with whatever physical conditions arise. Surgeons have observed that often there is need for less anaesthetics if the patient has been prepared mentally and spiritually for an operation. It has become the practice of many clergy to make every effort to visit a patient *prior* to an operation or some critical medical procedure, and the responses from patients are sufficiently positive to justify a continuation of this practice. Nevertheless, while this has been the common experience of caregivers, until recent years it has not received scientific examination. Lately attempts have been made to measure psycho-social interventions and their relationship to physical pain. A leader in this field is Ronald Melzack of the McGill University Faculty of Medicine in Montreal. He comments that there is "much convincing evidence that the pain experience is greatly influenced by expectations, suggestions, level of anxiety, and other psychologic variables."[17] He goes on to say, "The behaviours of patients who complain of pain is highly variable. The tissue damage that makes one patient a tragic invalid with constant pain may be regarded as a minor annoyance by another. Such differences emerge, at least in part, because persons differ in their perceptions of themselves and their environment, in their emotional and mood states, and in their learning histories."[18]

Because of all these variables we have to use considerable caution in assessing the extent of pain. The complaint of a patient could very easily be related to certain personality traits. Derek Doyle observes that "those who are primarily introverted experience more pain than those who are extroverts, but complain less about their suffering. Therefore, complained behaviour amongst patients is influenced to a considerable extent by this trait and reports of pain tend to be high among extroverts."[19]

Many other factors which affect the level of pain include interpersonal conflicts, threats of personal failure, environmental stress, decision conflicts, hysteria, depression, anxiety, attention-getting, and social abandonment. It has been pointed out that the social context in which the pain is experienced may alter its level of intensity. Barrie Cassileth, director of Psychosocial Programs at the University of Pennsylvania Cancer Center, has observed,

> Immediate context also influences response to the symptom of pain. More than 150 years ago it was attested that the extent of physical injury or wound bears little if any relationship to pain experienced. Beecher explored the issue in a controlled study of severe pain in civilian and wartime patients and concluded that "the concept underlying all experimental pain methods, that the more severe the pain stimuli to nerve endings, the more the pain, does not hold for pathological pain." Instead, differences in perceived pain between his two groups were attributable to the setting. On the battlefield a wound meant escape from the dangers and anxieties of war, and extreme physical damage was associated with relatively little pain. Similar civilian wounds, on the other hand, connoted disaster, and much higher levels of pain were found in this population. It is not difficult to generalize these findings to patients and to appreciate how setting influences sensitivity to pain and to other symptoms as well.[20]

In a very simple table R.G. Twycross of Churchill Hospital in Oxford, England, indicates how thresholds of pain can be lowered and raised.[21]

Factors Affecting Pain Threshold

Threshold lowered	*Threshold raised*
Discomfort	Relief of symptoms
Insomnia	Sleep
Fatigue	Rest
Anxiety	Sympathy
Fear	Understanding
Anger	Companionship
Sadness	Diversional activity
Depression	Reduction in anxiety
Boredom	Elevation of mood
Mental isolation	Analgesics
Social abandonment	Anxiolytics
	Antidepressants

Other methods for treating pain thresholds are being experimented by Ronald Melzack, including alpha-feed-back training, hypnosis, manipulation of breathing, and meditational techniques.[22] Although such experiments are in their infancy, they are contributing towards a greater knowledge of how psychosocial interventions can affect pain thresholds.

It could be argued that, whereas physical pain can be monitored in a scientific manner, it is impossible to incorporate the same methodology to measure spiritual interventions which, to all intents and purposes, are not quantifiable. And yet the research methods being adopted to measure the relationship between psycho-social interventions and the reduction of pain may also be applicable in the area of spirituality. It is fair to assume that, since the attendant results can be observed in a patient following psychological counselling, so the same information could be obtained after spiritual counselling. It is to be hoped that such research will be forthcoming.

This issue has been discussed in some detail in order to illustrate the interconnection between the various disciplines in the total care of the patient. Spirituality is no more an isolated field than any other discipline and should be understood as a complement to the work of other caregivers. This is not to enhance the credibility of spiritual care, but rather to emphasize that the total needs of the patient should be the object of care. If it is our responsibility in palliative care to provide the maximum relief of symptoms and ensure a quality of living, then that pain which militates against a quality of life must be alleviated by all possible means. It may very well be the case that spiritual care can make an important contribution towards this end.

Belief in the Next Life

Another area of spiritual concern raised by terminally ill patients is belief in the next life. In our present community of religious believers there has been a considerable change in the belief that life continues after death. The term *religious believers* refers to anyone who would claim to have some kind of religious affiliation or is at least willing to take the matter of religion seriously. Studies reveal that anywhere up to 30 per cent of practicing Christians in the main line churches do not believe, or else seriously doubt, the possibility of life after death.[23] A study done among young and well-educated respondents showed that they were quite indifferent about life after death, and 11 per cent definitely preferred that there not be a life after death.[24] And "the percentage of persons who report an increased belief in the afterlife following a life-threatening experience is less than 7 per cent."[25] This supports the statement made earlier that there are few death-bed conversions and that although a person may strengthen or integrate his or her religious beliefs we should not expect any radical changes.

There is also a declining interest in the next life among regular church members. If they are questioned why they attend church and make every effort to live a Christian life when they do not believe in a life after death, they reply that they live the good life because it is good in itself, and not because of any rewards in heaven. They believe that the Christian life enables them to realize their potential human nature and helps them find their place in society. Even if they were told with absolute certainty that there was no afterlife, they would still pattern their lives after the teaching of Christ. Such a response is in stark contrast to the more traditional teaching of the past, which preached the good life as a prerequisite for heaven. Such religious sentiments no longer captivate the minds of many religious people today.

But why has this change taken place? In recent years there has been a most significant change in the teaching about the nature of Christ, the nature of God, and the divine purpose for humanity. We have turned the emphasis away from the transcendence of God to a God who is very much involved in the affairs of this world, and we have concentrated our attention more on the humanity of Christ than his divinity. This has brought about a heightened concern for justice and good social order, greater efforts to improve the lot of human existence, and more emphasis on affirming the positive nature of humanity rather than revelling in its misdeeds. Some people have labelled this theological change as humanism, and this is a possible outcome of such thinking. Nevertheless, the change of emphasis could account for an increasing disinterest in the afterlife among Christian people. And it is possibly more accurate to call it "disinterest" rather than "complete disbelief."

There are, however, many people who reflect on the next life when they know that they are coming to the end of this life. Caregivers have noted that it is very common for patients to enquire about what happens after death. It may appear a little strange that in the midst of so much disbelief this issue should be raised so frequently. Part of the reason may be that we are often dealing with an older generation of people who have not shared the same doubts as the present generation. But whatever the reason, the fact that it is an important issue for many patients cannot be ignored.

It is also true that a large majority of those caring for the dying have a strong belief in the afterlife. One study, done by Anne Munley, estimates that 81 per cent believe that life continues after death, and 93 per cent of this group claim that it helps them in their work with terminally ill patients.[26] For them the next life is associated with peace and happiness, freedom from pain and worry, reunion with loved ones, and a life with God.

In the survey, there appears to be little mention about judgement and hell in the life after death. This again is not surprising, since there has been a marked change in our attitude towards the judgement of God and the possibility of eternal damnation.

From his own experience of talking about this issue with top-ranking clergy, Tom Harpur remarks that many "have now chopped hell altogether as an archaic concept unworthy of the loving God declared by Christ. It is still part of the theological dogma, but in practice it is ignored. The prevailing thought is that everyone will be "saved" eventually. Even those main-liners who cling to the doctrine of hell do so with some embarrassment combined with a great deal of compassion."[27]

There are, of course, those who believe it is their mission in life to wage a campaign against the powers of the devil. The sole purpose of their message is to rescue mankind from the torments of hell. While it may very well be true that a man will find himself in hell, I believe he is not put there by God, but rather by himself. Support for this interpretation comes from the parable of the rich man and Lazarus. In the parable both men die. The uncaring, selfish rich man finds himself in hell, but Lazarus is pictured lying in the bosom of Abraham. While Lazarus enjoys the loving company of Abraham, who traditionally symbolizes the people of Israel, the rich man is pictured bereft of any loving community around him. The imagery is made even more poignant in that the rich man is able to see what Lazarus is enjoying, but cannot get to it himself. Perhaps hell is finally recognizing the beauty and goodness of love, but not being able to receive or partake of it. A very simple definition of hell is going to heaven and not liking it.

There is little more that one can say about the next life. We cannot speak with absolute certainty concerning further spiritual attainment, although it would seem consistent with a loving God that all those who have died in younger years, those who have had the misfortune of enduring a handicap in this life, will be given the opportunity of continued spiritual growth. But this can only be a hopeful expectation. What we can be assured of, through our faith in Christ, is that we will not be aimless spirits drifting through empty space, nor will we enter the next life like a drop of water falling into the ocean only to disappear and be absorbed into the Godhead. Rather, we will enter a life of community where we will learn to love perfectly and be perfectly loved. Those who have tasted some of this love here on earth will know, even through a glass darkly, what to expect later. Sometimes such knowledge is only experienced in the last days

of life when a person is surrounded by caregivers who are truly
trying to exemplify God's love. But it is this kind of loving which
will remove fear and help a person make a peaceful transition
into the life to come.

The Significance of the Resurrection

It is at this point that we should consider the significance of the
resurrection of Christ, both as it applies to the next life and to
the life we live here and now. It would not be particularly useful
within the context of this book to indulge in a long detailed dissertation about the historic value of the resurrection. It is sufficient to say that the bodily resurrection of Christ as an historic
event is an important part of the Christian tradition, and that it
contains a significant symbolic message for the Christian believer.
At the same time I would hasten to add that speaking of the resurrection as the final day of judgement, when graves will open and
the dead will be raised in bodily form to meet their God, is not,
in my opinion, a particularly relevant interpretation of this event.

The bodily resurrection of Christ signifies that in the next life
we are promised an existence which will involve personal recognition within a communal life. Even as our bodies now are the
vehicles through which we are able to communicate and express
our personal identity, and as a result build community through
personal relationships, so in the next life we are promised some
kind of "spiritual body" which will enable us to continue our
spiritual development within a communal environment. Our
minds cannot really comprehend what lies beyond this, and when
we try to describe it, we inevitably resort to poetic or symbolic
language. We simply have to be content with the promise which
God has given us in Christ.

There is at least another point we can learn from the resurrection event. It is important to remember that the resurrection was
preceded by the crucifixion. The promise of new life was preceded
by death. This would seem to indicate that new life, in any form,
can be acquired only when a death is involved. And this is borne
out by life's experiences.

We cannot deny the fact that both physically and spiritually our
lives continually have the potential for regeneration. Our lives
are constantly changing. We receive new insights, undertake new

tasks, establish new relationships, and develop new skills. These could be classifed as resurrection experiences, because it is through them that we receive new life.)At the same time we have to be prepared for an experience of death if this new life is to come into being. This rhythm of new life emerging out of death has been described in this way.

> Thinking of this in terms of our personal growth, we might illustrate these "death" and "new life" experiences in this way: a child must die to crawling in order to live for walking; a person must die to particular relationships in one family in order to live for a new relationship in marriage; a person must die to another in bereavement in order to live for a new set of relationships with others; a person must die to one job in order to live for a new style of work; a person must die to work in order to live for retirement. These are the "little deaths" constituting the variety of changes we must experience in order that growth and new life may come into being. It would seem that, as we face these "little deaths" constructively in the midst of life, we become better prepared to face the death of our physical bodies and the new spiritual life promised to us.[28]

This view of life and death has been beautifully summarized in the words of H.A. Williams. "If we are ready for life in the sense of being open to its power and possibilities, then we are also ready for death. If we are aware of resurrection in the present, then we shall not be overconcerned about resurrection in the future."[29]

Perhaps people would have less difficulty acting responsibly at the end of life if they had dealt responsibly with these "minor deaths" during their lifetime. This does not mean that it is possible to be completely prepared for death, but it is possible that we can understand and ease the passage if we have attuned ourselves into life's rhythm of death and resurrection.

Unfortunately, this is not an easy task to accomplish under present conditions. We have quite rightly been called an acquisitive society, one that is eager to acquire and loathe to relinquish. We accumulate a wealth of things, experiences, acquaintances, skills, knowledge, material possessions — all of which can overburden us unless we are capable of relinquishing the old in order to acquire the new. We are constantly challenged to reassess the lifestyle we are carrying with us and, if necessary, die to one thing in order to live for something else. Death should not symbolize past failure but rather future hope. This kind of spiritual interpretation of death can give meaning and purpose to the event, and so enable people to reach a state of peace and hope all through life.

The Quest for Immortality

In the course of history there have been many myths and fables about humanity's quest for immortality. The stories describing man's discovery of some idyllic Shangri-la or the fountain of youth abound in English literature. One can assume that underlying these stories is a secret yearning for immortality, and even though it may be presented as a wishful fantasy, the fact remains that it betrays an avoidance of death. It is interesting to consider what it would be like if such a dream came true.

There are other stories which describe the situation differently. In Homer's *Odyssey*, Ulysses meets the sea princess Calypso who is destined to live forever in this world. She expresses acute envy of Ulysses because some day he will die. In *Gulliver's Travels* we are told that Gulliver was overjoyed to learn that he would meet a race of people among whom certain individuals were chosen at birth to live forever. He expects them to be the happiest people in the world but discovers that they are the most miserable. They grow old and weak, losing all sense of time and purpose. It has for them become a fate worse than death.

The historical veracity of such fables is irrelevant. What is true is our inability to accept death as a part of life. We do not like facing the end of anything. But what would it be like to have the gift of composing music and never be allowed to write the final chords? What would it be like to be a brilliant author and never be given permission to write the last chapter? We would find this intolerable. I am reminded of my father's comment when I asked him how he felt after he had completed a painting. He acknowledged that it was a good feeling because he could then enjoy facing a new blank canvas. To live in a world without "endings" would be equivalent to an existence without any meaning and fulfilment. It is a rhythm we must all capture as we proceed with our spiritual journey.

Notes

1 Susan J. Quinn, "Elderly in Hospice," *The American Journal of Hospice Care* 1 (1984), p. 29.

2 John K. Swift, "The Chaplain's Role in Care for the Dying: toward a new understanding," *Canadian Medical Association Journal* 115 (July 17, 1976), p. 182.

3 *Ibid.*, p. 182.

4 Harold S. Kushner, *When Bad Things Happen to Good People* (New York: Avon Books, 1981), p. 3.

5 John D. Shanahan, "The role of the clergy in the care of seriously ill patients," *Annals New York Academy of Sciences* 164 (1969), p. 750.

6 R. Lamerton, "Religion and the Care of the Dying," *Nursing Times* 69 (January 18, 1973), p. 89.

7 Glanville Williams, *The Sanctity of Life and the Criminal Law* (London: Faber and Faber, 1958), p. 280.

8 Harold S. Kushner, *op. cit*, p. 43.

9 Cicely Saunders, ed., *Beyond All Pain* (London: S.P.C.K., 1983), p. 33.

10 Viktor Frankl, *Man's Search for Meaning* (New York: Pocket Books, 1963), p. 105.

11 *Ibid.*, p. 179.

12 Christine Allen, "Bridging the Gulf of Meaning," *The Royal Victoria Hospital Manual on Palliative/Hospice Care* (New York: Arno Press, 1980), p. 236.

13 Matthew Fox, *Whee! We, wee All the Way Home* (North Carolina: Consortium Books, 1976), p. 68.

14 Cicely Saunders, "I was sick and you visited me," *In the Service of Medicine — A Quarterly Paper* 42 (July 1965), p. 2.

15 *Ibid.*, p. 2.

16 Shirley du Boulay, *Cicely Saunders* (London: Hodder and Stoughton, 1984), p. 175.

17 Ronald Melzack, "Psychologic Aspects of Pain," *Postgraduate Medicine* 53 (May 1973), p. 69.

18 *Ibid.*, p. 70.

19 Derek Doyle, ed., *Palliative Care: The Management of Far-Advanced Illness* (London: Croom Helm, 1984), p. 246.

20 Barrie R. Cassileth, "Hospice and the biopsychosocial model of health care," *The American Journal of Hospice Care* 1 (1984), p. 19.

21 R.G. Twycross, "Ethical and Clinical Aspects of Pain Treatment in Cancer Patients," *Acta Anaesth. Scand.* 74, 83–90 (1982), p. 89.

22 Ronald Melzack, *op. cit.*, p. 73–74.

23 Reginald Bibby, *Windsor Star* (April 2, 1983).

24 Victor Marshall, *Last Chapters* (California: Brooks/Cole Publishing Company, 1980), p. 178.

25 *Ibid.*, p. 178.

26 Anne Munley, *The Hospice Alternative* (New York: Basic Books Inc. Publisher, 1983), p. 252.

27 Tom Harpur, *Harpur's Heaven and Hell* (Toronto: Oxford University Press, 1983), p. 232.

28 Lawrence Whytehead and Paul Chidwick, editors, *Dying, considerations concerning the passage from life to death* (Toronto: Anglican Book Centre, 1980), p. 61.

29 H.A. Williams, *True Resurrection* (New York: Harper and Row, 1974), p. 177.

The Responsibility to Care

The current enthusiasm to care more effectively for the dying has swept through many countries in the world. It is undoubtedly a valid concern. But it is also valid to ask, What is the reason for this concern? It has all the earmarks of a twentieth-century phenomenon appearing on the human scene as the latest popular fad. Everyone is climbing on the bandwagon to be part of this new health-care service. How do we account for all this enthusiasm?

We know that people have been dying since the world began. We also know that they have been cared for by their families or by the available medical personnel of their day. There have even been religious orders established specifically to care for the dying, and this goes back to the medieval period. The Hospice Movement is not a new invention. And it is most unfortunate that those who have become involved in this work sometimes appear as the enlightened ones who have suddenly realized that the dying need to be cared for. Such an image can be very threatening to those already working in the health-care field, and we must make every effort to dispel such an image, simply because it is grossly incorrect.

There are reasons for the ascendancy of hospice care, reasons which are unique to our time. The first is our technical ability to keep people with life-threatening illnesses alive longer, thereby giving us more time to provide effective care. The second is our increased knowledge about their physical, psychological, social, and spiritual needs. We have dared to bring the subject of death out into the open, and we have engaged in honest communication with those who are facing death. But all of this is still not sufficient to account for the overwhelming interest to care more effectively for the dying.

The most singular and innovative aspect of this work in our day is that the findings have been documented. And the reporting has been done in a way which can claim medical and scientific respectability, without being erudite and incomprehensible to the average person. These findings have not been filed in abstract medical journals but have been presented in a popular form, so that the ordinary person can understand what the needs are and make some effort to respond to them. This constitutes the uniqueness of hospice care in the twentieth century and accounts in large measure for its rapid growth over the past two decades.

One of the most important things we have learned from our dialogue with the terminally ill is their fear of abandonment. We know that there will always be people who fear death, and it is certainly not uncommon for people to fear the way in which they will die. But the most common fear is that someone is going to pin a sign on their door saying, "Nothing more can be done," and then all they can do is to lie back and watch the retreat begin. Unfortunately this does take place and often in a number of subtle ways.

A patient once said to me that, when he had been told that he had a limited life expectancy, he was immediately admitted into hospital, and every day his family would come and visit him. When they left they would always give him a kiss and a hug. And then he said, "Something strange happened after a couple of months. When they left they stopped giving me a kiss and a hug. They just squeezed my hand." And in a very dejected tone of voice, he added, "Do you know what they do now when they leave? They wave at the door." A very subtle and no doubt unconscious form of abandonment, but the message was clear to the patient.

Very recently an experiment was performed with children who had life-threatening illnesses. The children were given a model box of the hospital room, and in the box there was a bed, side table, cupboard, and door with miniature figures representing the nurse, the doctor, and various members of the family. The children were told to put the figures anywhere they wanted, and if they decided to move them around they could do so. It was discovered that, as the children got closer to the point of death, the figures moved closer to the door. The children were not capable of verbalizing what was happening, but that feeling of abandonment was very real to them.

Other experiments have been done which indicate that nurses may take longer to answer the call of a terminally ill patient than a patient who will get well, that doctors often visit less frequently, that visits become briefer, and that conversations take place in a hushed and perfunctory manner. Such revelations have led people to try to redress the situation, and to provide patients with more people giving more time.

In the majority of instances the people who have engaged in this work have had some personal experience with death, either of a friend or of a family member. This is particularly true when we consider those who have volunteered for this work. In some cases a person has felt inadequate in dealing with the death, and has been concerned to rectify the situation. In other cases the experience was positive and the individual has recognized the value of effective interventions with such patients. But whatever the reason, there is a growing awareness that not enough people are giving sufficient time to provide adequate care. This is a very significant reason for the present-day concern to be more responsible in meeting the needs of the terminally ill.

Opportunities for the Patient To Be a Responsible Caregiver

Unfortunately something else has happened which has made this kind of health care a little one-sided. Our new insights have blinded us to another aspect of caring which is equally important. In our enthusiasm to provide better care for the dying we have not paid much attention to the opportunities for the dying to care more effectively for the living. To some extent our concern for the needs of the dying has resulted in caring them to death. We have, on many occasions, over-extended our care at the expense of denying people the opportunity to fulfil some of their own personal responsibilities at this time.

Understandably, we do this with the best of intentions. After all, should we not feel sorry for those about to face the end of life? We want to do everything we can to make their remaining days and weeks free of any worries or difficulties. And to suggest that we should encourage them to act responsibly may seem somewhat callous and cruel. Is this not making too heavy a demand on a person facing the end of life? However, fulfilling responsibilities is a significant part of living and should not be denied the dying.

Laurie O'Brien, the director of the Palliative Care Unit at St.

Clare's Mercy Hospital in St. John's, Newfoundland, pointed out how important it was to work with the family and help them realize that the patient was still alive. She and her staff had discovered that families can become so over-protective that they rob the patient of any further effective living. The patient is treated as a docile and helpless individual with nothing further to offer the world. This is certainly not a healthy message to convey to any person, let alone someone who is dying.

We have seen that it is common for people with a limited life expectancy to look inward and make a personal assessment of their life with the hope of finding what has been of value. This enables them to give meaning to their life and so provides them with a sense of peace and fulfilment. Such persons are, of course, living in the past, and, while this may be understandable, it will inevitably have the effect of divorcing that person from any life in the future, limited though it may be. While a life review is very important for a patient, it can have the effect of militating against possible accomplishments in the time remaining. But why is this so important?

We have seen that one significant aspect of human nature is the ability to make decisions. People have the freedom to choose what they will say and do in life. When they make choices which either benefit themselves or those around them, they can achieve a sense of self-worth, knowing that their lives are of value to themselves and others. But if someone refuses or is denied the opportunity to make decisions, then that person has given up, or has been robbed of, that very significant aspect of human nature. By helping people realize that their decision making is important, we are conveying the message that they are still needed, that as human beings they are still worth something in this world.

There is another reason why we should encourage the dying to engage in responsible decision making. Whatever we may believe about a life after death in general, most of us have some concern about what people will think of *our* life after death in particular. How will they remember us? Will these be happy memories to soothe the pains of separation? What sort of parting gift will we leave this world? It would be sad if these memories included unanswered questions, unresolved differences, feelings of guilt, financial confusion, or various kinds of other unfinished business. Regrettably, more of this happens than we realize.

In an extensive study of bereavement among widows, Mary Vachon discovered that sometimes less than 30 per cent of the couples engaged in any meaningful discussion about the impending death. A far greater percentage chose to avoid the subject. And she concludes that much of the popular death and dying literature has apparently had little effect on the populace.[1] In a survey done in Great Britain, Geoffrey Gorer found that not one of the 30 widows he interviewed had been able to discuss what was happening to her husband before his death.[2] He discovered considerable regret and bitterness among the bereaved. This absence of communication is an unfortunate legacy to leave behind. And it raises the question as to who should be responsible for initiating better communication.

We can make the assumption that the onus should fall on the caregiver or a family member. No doubt this can happen, but often the caregiver becomes protective and shields the patient from issues which may cause further discomfort. Is it not possible to consider that the patient could give permission for such communication to begin? This is only one aspect of a patient's opportunity to care, but it can have a tremendous effect on both patients and family members alike. Cicely Saunders comments, ''I have often seen patients where death has been greatly eased by the knowledge that they were doing something for their families right to the end.''[3] It is these kinds of opportunities which we need to encourage.

It is interesting to note how certain biblical figures have responded to approaching death. When Abraham was about to die, his last act was to secure a wife for his son so that God's promise to build a mighty nation from the seed of Abraham would be fulfilled (Genesis 24:1–9). The aged Jacob, nearly blind, gathered his family around him and bestowed special blessings on each of his sons. He provided them all with hope: ''I am dying. God will be with you and will bring you back to the land of your fathers'' (Genesis 48:21). In the same way, when Moses was about to die, he showed no resentment that he was denied the opportunity to enter the Promised Land, but gave people hope for the future. His parting words: ''The Lord has told me that I may not cross the Jordan. The Lord your God will cross over at your head'' (Deuteronomy 31:2–3). As the prophet Elijah was preparing to leave this world, he was accompanied by his companion Elisha.

When the end came Elijah said to Elisha, "Tell me what I can do for you before I am taken from you." Elisha replied, "Let me inherit a double share of your spirit," and the wish was granted (2 Kings 2:2-3).

In the New Testament there are similar examples of people acting responsibly in the face of death. When John the Baptist was facing execution in prison, he challenged his followers to clarify in their minds what the ministry of Jesus was all about, thereby giving them permission to transfer their allegiance to him. Both Paul and the author of the Book of Revelation continued to correspond with the churches while they were imprisoned and expecting death at any moment. And our Lord himself, in spite of his suffering, offered forgiveness to his enemies, gave hope to a thief who was sharing the same fate, and made provision for the care of his mother. All these are examples of people facing death and yet recognizing the opportunities to care for the living.

But it would be wrong just to single out the great heroes of the past or, for that matter, of the Judaeo-Christian tradition. Victor Marshall cites the custom among the Kalai tribe of New Britain in Melanesia. "When the Kalai realize that death is approaching, they try to ward it off. The time thus gained is spent bringing social relationships to a close. In the idealized good death, the dying person called all his kinsmen to gather round him, disposed of his possessions after repaying the obligations owed by him and forgiving any obligations of others to him, and then informed those gathered that it was time for him to die."[4] Similar traditions were quite common among different races prior to the thirteenth century. Philippe Aries describes this much earlier attitude towards death in this way. "Sorrow was expressed that life must end, one's relations with others was made right, and then attention was turned to God. All this was organized *by* rather than *for* the individual, and it involved family, including children, friends, and neighbors."[5]

Archbishop Donald Arden of Central Africa related a personal experience concerning the death of an African Christian. "The death of the old is quite different, and the domestic theology of the living-dead draws on a wisdom that the West has lost. In Swaziland I spent a night with the medical assistant of a government clinic, who was also the leader of a little Christian congregation. Another guest was his father, a gentle, happy man in his late sixties, who lived eighty miles away. On my next monthly round I was shocked to be told by my friend that his father had just died at the family home. I expressed surprise, since he had seemed to be in excellent health, and asked of what he had died. 'Nothing, it was just his time. We are four children in the family, so he came to stay with each of us for a week and talk and play with all his grandchildren, and to say good-bye. He reached home last week, and now he has gone. It is good.' "[6]

These examples illustrate that acting responsibly in the face of death is not the monopoly of any particular race or culture. It is an activity which is basic to human nature and speaks about an aspect of spirituality that lies within all of us. What we need to consider now is how a patient can exercise such spirituality among the variety of caregivers who surround him.

Opportunities for the Dying To Care for the Living

A patient can care for friends and family by trying to alleviate grief and guilt. Feelings of grief do not begin only after the death occurs, but are usually there in some anticipatory form as soon as it is realized that a person's life expectancy is limited. And it is not only the next of kin who experience grief; the patient is also aware of pending separation. On many occasions it is only when the patient verbalizes the grief that permission is given to the family to share their own feelings. This release can go a long way towards alleviating the pain of separation after the death occurs.

It is also extremely hard to assist people to work through the grieving process if there exists an abnormal amount of guilt about the former relationship. There are times when no amount of counselling has any effect. The person is really wanting absolution from the departed, and the opportunity has passed. This does not mean that the situation is hopeless. It is just that guilt seems to paralyze the grieving process. And if there had been better communication, the process could have been facilitated.

Feelings of guilt can arise in a number of ways. The bereaved person may feel that he or she could have done more during the illness; there could be some unresolved differences which needed to be reconciled; in the case of a long and painful terminal illness the next of kin may have secretly wished for that person's death; there may be times when the spouse feels angry for having been left alone — all of which can instigate feelings of guilt. During the bereavement period people may feel guilty about the absence of tears; they may feel it is a sign of unfaithfulness if they begin to value other relationships; they may have feelings of anger and hostility against God for allowing such a tragedy to take place (and the guilt arising from these feelings may account for the large number of people who disengage themselves from any religious affiliation during the bereavement period); they may recall things done or left undone which can no longer be rectified; they may develop anxiety and guilt over various decisions which have to be made in order to settle the estate.

It is very sad and frustrating to see a bereaved person trying to read the mind of the departed, as he or she makes funeral arrangements, disposes of belongings, sells the car, decides whether to continue membership in an organization which they both shared, or whether it would be fitting to participate in a little enjoyable entertainment? There is this continual preoccupation with the question, Is this the way he or she would want me to do it? How much mystery and confusion would be avoided if there had been the opportunity to openly face the issues together? How much guilt would be removed if there had been a more concerted effort to reconcile the past. As Cicely Saunders so rightly says, "Memories of a time that enabled old guilts to be resolved and that changed the very nature of the past by its reconciliations will transform the slow process of mourning."[7]

As an example of how grief and reconciliations can be resolved by the dying person, it might be appropriate to recount an event that took place during the death of my wife's mother. She was dying of cancer, and her last request was to see all her grandchildren once more. Over a period of weeks they arrived from different parts of the country to be with her and say their farewells. One of the grandchildren, on the evening prior to her returning home, broke down in tears and said that she would not go up to the hospital that evening. She was quite sure that she would cry, say all the wrong things, and be an embarrassment to everyone in the room. She knew that she might feel very guilty later if she did not go, but she continued to be fearful about not being able to control her feelings. We finally agreed to go to the hospital and while she waited in the corridor I went into the room alone and asked everyone to leave. Mother looked weary and was having some discomfort. She was also a little indignant about losing all her visitors. I said to her: "Mother, you have a granddaughter out in the hall and she is being torn apart because she is saying good-bye for the last time. She is afraid of crying and making a fool of herself. There is only one person who can do anything for her — and that's you." The response was immediate. She sat up in bed, and with complete disregard for her discomfort, she said, "Send that girl in. I know how to deal with her." Then followed the tears, the forgivenesses, the expressions of love, the joy and laughter about past events — and this was Granny's parting gift to that child. She gave permission for that young child to be herself and resolve her grief. When they parted that girl carried away a gift she will never forget. And the message to Granny was more than just a challenge to fulfil a family responsibility; it was also a clear message that she was still needed. It was an appeal to her spiritual nature, and she readily responded.

Often patients have been deliberately challenged to fulfil a certain task, and have risen magnificently to the occasion. Especially I remember some incidents related to the founding of the Hospice of Windsor. There was much that we had to learn about providing effective care, and we thought that the best teachers would be the patients themselves. We approached Flora with our plans. She was enthusiastic and very detailed in her suggestions about those things which were important to her — the need for open visitation, the personally prepared meals, the presence of someone during the night. She even told us to get rid of our smocks (a bilious yellow colour). We needed her advice and she responded. As we developed our public relations with the media, we needed someone who would be prepared to tell her story on television. We were given the name of Eileen, whose life expectancy had been extended by three years. Her determination to live every day as fully as possible, and not give in to despair and self-pity, had made this possible. She told her story, and not only assisted our cause but also gave us a teaching mechanism for our volunteers. Also we asked Rita if she might speak to a newspaper reporter about her impressions of the palliative care we were offering. In a very lucid and forthright manner she shared her ideas for two or three hours and provided insights which only a person in her situation could do. That was her parting gift; she died two days later.

There are numerous examples of how individuals have responded to a need, and as a result have helped to enhance faith in others, remove the fear of death, stimulate a love for life, provide courage, and above all enable others to focus on the real values in life. Their willingness to respond indicates how important it is for them to feel needed.

Other opportunities for the patient to care lie in the area of establishing better communication with medical personnel. A complaint we sometimes hear from patients is that no one ever tells them anything. The patient may feel that he or she has been surrounded by a conspiracy of silence. The whole matter of information giving has been hotly debated over the years. In some studies it has been discovered that 90 per cent of cancer patients want to know their diagnosis, whereas 60 per cent to 90 per cent of their physicians advise against telling them.[8] Such studies might suggest that the doctor is an aloof and uncaring individual with no concern for the thoughts and feelings of his patients. Obviously this is a rash assumption. But how do we account for such different attitudes towards communication?

The first thing to recognize is that, generally speaking, patients do not expect the doctor to make mistakes. How many times have patients lost confidence in their doctor because of a changed diagnosis? As a result a doctor will be very cautious about what she says because she knows that she cannot go back on her word without suffering the consequences. Furthermore, to tell people that they have a fatal illness can be a wrenching experience. It is not easy to convey this kind of information and then calmly walk out the door. The doctor may not be trained as a counsellor, nor does she always have time to help the patient come to grips with this emotional crisis. She may also be asking herself some very vital questions: ''Does this patient really want to talk about his condition? How much information can he take? Will he resent me intruding into this part of his life which he may want to deny? Will he become more depressed and angry? These can be very agonizing questions for any caregiver. How then is it possible to develop better communication between the patient and doctor?

In an article called "What a Dying Man Taught a Doctor about Caring" Caroline Driver cites a particular case where there was a complete wall of detachment between the doctor and the patient.

Now, at 34, Bob was dying. Even though he was to make comeback after comeback and neither of us ever really gave up hope, he knew the odds. What's more, the staff knew he knew. Yet he might have been a piece of protoplasm with a serial number; the young doctor simply marked the chart and started to leave. But at this point Bob stopped him.

"Just a moment, Doctor . . ."

The doctor turned in surprise at the directness of Bob's tone.

"Doctor," Bob continued evenly, "I don't . . . like you."

The startled physician reacted with arrogance. "Mr. Driver," he snapped back, "I'm a doctor here. What's more, I'm *your* doctor."

"Then you know I'm fighting for my life," Bob said. "So why do you come in with negativeness and coldness. Why?"

Shaken, the young M.D. sat down. "I'm sorry," he said, "I don't like to be that way with people. I just find it hard to reach out the way you do. Sometimes I wonder why I'm this way myself."

With that the two men talked for nearly an hour. When the doctor finally departed they had begun a genuine friendship.[9]

It goes without saying that this is not a typical incident but the dramatic nature of the case highlights certain issues. The patient reached out to resolve a situation. Bob realized that he was the only person capable of reconciling an intolerable relationship. It was certainly risky, but it does illustrate that there can be a place for the patient to take the initiative in achieving better communication between himself and the caregivers around him. It would greatly improve any situation if the doctor knew just how well the patient was able to cope with unpleasant news. It is very important to assess a person's receptivity before providing certain kinds of information; and unless one is an astute counsellor, it becomes a sort of guessing game. Consequently, the doctor would welcome reassurance from the patient and the family that they are ready to hear about the diagnosis.

Bob also reached out to the nursing staff. "Later on there was a nurse we thought was unfriendly till we found out it was because Bob resembled a brother who had died. She had to fight back the tears every time she came near us. Bob encouraged her to sit down and let the tears flow. That broke the tension, and she relaxed with us from then on. Another nurse happened to like us but feared being accused of playing favourites if she got too chummy. After Bob got her to laughing at herself a bit, she said, 'Oh to hell with what people think!' and sat down too."[10] Many of us would be very surprised if we knew why people withdraw from tragic situations. It is sometimes the patient who can help people resolve these anxieties.

Another group which sometimes needs help is the clergy. By virtue of their training they are pictured (or they picture themselves) as the people with all the answers to difficult questions. One of the pitfalls which most clergy fall into is to make a visitation with a prescribed agenda. The clergy then dominate the visits and come away unscathed. Their fear is that they will be asked questions for which they do not have satisfactory answers, and this sense of helplessness makes the caregivers feel most uncomfortable. But helplessness is not such a bad feeling if it leaves you open to the needs of the patient. When patients recognize your honesty and see that you have allowed yourself to become vulnerable, very often they will reassure you that they do not expect the clergy to be the repository of all the truth. And within this kind of interaction the patient finds an opportunity to care for us. It becomes yet another instance when the patient receives the message that he or she is still needed.

In this chapter we have emphasized the importance of recognizing those situations where patients may have the opportunity to act in a responsible and caring manner to those around them. One way to prevent this from happening is to try to do everything for them. We have already seen how families can become over-protective. We would do well to have a little more respect for the capabilities and intelligence of the terminally ill. We must not underestimate their mental or spiritual capacities. They are struggling for value and meaning, and any indication that they are needed will be recognized immediately. The human personality has a way of drawing on inner resources for any kind of meaningful activity. It is up to us to allow it to happen. This is one very important way of allowing patients to engage in a significant spiritual activity.

St. Christopher, the saint whom Cicely Saunders followed so closely, dedicated himself to carrying pilgrims across the water and discovered that his burden was in fact the Christ child. Caregivers who assist people in their final efforts to act as responsible individuals, will see them reaching towards maturity in Christ, and in doing so they will share the burden of St. Christopher.

Notes

1   Mary Vachon, "The final illness in cancer; the widow's perspective," *Canadian Medical Association Journal* 117 (November 19, 1977), p. 1152.
2   Cicely Saunders, "Death and Responsibility," *Psychiatric Opinion* (August 1966), p. 32.
3   *Ibid.*, p. 31.
4   Victor Marshall, *Last Chapters, A Sociology of Aging and Dying* (California: Brook/Cole Publishing Company, 1980), p. 34.
5   *Ibid.*, p. 44.
6   Donald Coggan, "Moral and Spiritual Aspects," The Edwin Stevens Lecture, *Proceedings of the Royal Society of Medicine* 70 (1977), p. 79.
7   Cicely Saunders, *op. cit.*, p. 34.
8   Charles A. Garfield, *Psychosocial Care of the Dying Patient* (New York: McGraw-Hill Book Company, 1978), p. 108.
9   *Ibid.*; p. 73.
10 *Ibid.*, p. 76.

Phenomenal Experiences —
Spiritual, Psychological or Both?

Certain inexplicable experiences sometimes occur among those who are approaching death. There have been hundreds of instances where people claim that they have temporarily left this life and have entered a higher state of consciousness, or believe that they have come in touch with another form of reality. These experiences can take a variety of forms and can come upon a person at any moment. The particular phenomena that will concern us in this chapter are those experienced at the point of death, either through some sudden accident or in the course of a lingering dying process, such as leaving one's body and yet being aware of one's surroundings, leaving this world temporarily and supposedly getting a glimpse of a reality beyond this life (sometimes known as life-after-death experiences), being visited or being in communication with the departed, or having visions or dreams which might be considered as premonitions of death. Even though the experiences vary in form, they all suggest a reality other than that which we know in our space-time environment. Whether or not these events are subjective projections or objective realities outside the individual, they are very real to those who have experienced them, and for this reason, they need to be addressed.

There has been a greater public awareness of these phenomena through the recent publications of such people as Raymond A. Moody, *Life After Life*, Karlis Osis and Erlendur Haraldsson, *At the Hour of Death*, and Elisabeth Kübler-Ross, *On Children and Death*.[1] But this should in no way lead us to believe that the experiences are unique to the twentieth century. In an article written sixteen years ago, Rosalind Heywood suggests that such phenomena are more numerous than commonly assumed. She says, ''There are a few hints, however, that it may be less rare than is assumed. Apart from the reports of it amassed by such bodies as The British and American Societies for Psychical Research and continental researchers, cases are quoted and discussed in books written since the last war by Stephen Findlay, Marghanita Laski, Professors R.C. Zaehnew and W.T. Stace, and Drs. Raynor Johnson, F.C. Happold, and Louisa Rhine. Dr. Robert Crookall has collected reports of hundreds of such experiences and classified them according to family resemblances, and a well-known American sociologist, the late Professor Hornell Hart, made a long term study of them.''[2]

I dare say that few, if any, of the names mentioned above, will be recognized by the reader; unlike Moody and Kübler-Ross, their findings have been reported in philosophical and medical journals. The only point I am making is that such phenomena have been happening for ages and must not be considered unique to our generation. Indeed, we can even go back to the experience of Plotinus (c.204–270) ''Many a time it happened to me — lifted out of the body into myself, becoming external to all other things, beholding a marvellous beauty, assured of community with the highest order, acquiring identity with the divine . . . . Yet there comes the moment of descent.''[3]

It would be easy to associate these experiences with people who have a somewhat disturbed psychological background. Some critics might consider such experiences to be hallucinations resulting from a neurotic disorder. Consequently, we may tend to be prejudicial about the type of person who is prone to such phenomena. And yet we would do well to remember that we have autobiographical evidence of out-of-the-body experiences from such people as Wordsworth, Emily Bronte, George Eliot, George Meredith, Tennyson, Arnold Bennett, D.H. Lawrence, Virginia Woolf, Warner Allen, Bernard Berenson, John Buchan, William Gerhardi, Arthur Koestler, and Ernest Hemingway. This, in itself, does not prove such experiences to be valid. It is not impossible for the finest minds in the world to have hallucinations. It is likely, however, that such experiences are not the monopoly of any one kind of person, and that we should take them seriously.

Examples of Out-of-Body Experiences

It might be helpful if we quoted some examples of these experiences, over and above what we have been hearing from those dealing with terminally ill patients. The following occurred to a very fit mountaineer during his struggle to climb back to safety, after having fallen over the edge of a precipice. He wrote, "I found myself hanging on to a rope a few feet below the crest of the ridge. I turned, scratched at the rocks and clawed my way back. I had fallen altogether about 20 feet and the rope . . . had held . . . . During the time I was doing this a curious rigidity of tension gripped my whole being, mental and physical . . . . It was an overwhelming sensation and quite outside my experience. It was as if all life's focus were in process of undergoing some fundamental evolutionary change, the change called death . . . . I know now that death is not to be feared, it is a surpreme experience, the climax, not the anti-climax of life. For how long I experienced this crescendo of power I cannot say. Time no longer existed as time . . . . Then suddenly this feeling was superceded by a feeling of complete indifference and detachment, detachment as to what was happening or likely to happen to the body. I seemed to stand aside from my body. I was not falling for the reason that I was not in a dimension where it was possible to fall. I, that is my consciousness, was apart from my body and not in the least concerned with what was befalling it."[4]

Another person had a similar experience on the battlefield. "During the war in the Western Desert, I was knocked unconscious by a bomb blast and had a peculiar sensation of being out of my body viewing the scene from a point about 20 feet above the ground . . . . I could hear the aircraft as it came in on another attack and the voices of my companions. I could see the dust clearing away from the explosion and my own body lying there on the ground . . . . I remember the thought, 'I've got to get back', and then . . . I was back in my body consciously trying to force my eyes open. An odd thing was that, although I could hear perfectly while I was unconscious and could tell my comrades what they had said during that period, when I recovered consciousness I was stone deaf and remained so for two weeks afterwards . . . . This experience has convinced me that there is a part of the person that survives after death . . . . I am certain that when I do eventually die, or rather when my body dies, part of me will carry on, to where or to do what I do not know."[5]

A somewhat typical account is given by a woman who suffered from a heart attack. She recalls, "About a year ago, I was admitted to the hospital with heart trouble, and the next morning, lying in a hospital bed, I began to have a very severe pain in my chest.

I pushed the button beside the bed to call for the nurses, and they came in and started working on me. I was quite uncomfortable lying on my back so I turned over, and as I did I quit breathing and my heart stopped beating. Just then, I heard the nurse shout, 'Code pink! Code pink!' As they were saying this, I could feel myself moving out of my body . . . . Then, I started rising upward, slowly . . . . I watched them revive me from up there! My body was lying down there stretched out on the bed, in plain view, and they were all standing around it. I heard one nurse say, 'Oh, my God! She's gone!', while another one leaned down to give me mouth to mouth resuscitation . . . . As I saw them below beating on my chest and rubbing my arms and legs, I thought, 'Why are they going to so much trouble? I'm just fine now.' "[6]

Some people find these experiences frightening, but for the most part there is a feeling of euphoria, a contentment, and an unwillingness to return to their former reality. People speak as if they have passed into another dimension and as a result find it difficult to describe their experience in our three-dimensional terminology. In many accounts, the experients wax poetic and this in turn tends to give the account an air of unreality. If we were to try to summarize a typical experience, one which contains the most frequently mentioned characteristics, the description by Hans Küng would suit our purposes. He writes and quotes Raymond Moody:

The typical case, which admittedly is never completely verified, but of which important elements are found . . . might be described more or less on these lines: When a person lies dying and reaches the climax of his bodily agony, he can hear the doctor declaring him dead. Then he hears an unpleasant sound, a piercing ringing or buzzing. At the same time he feels that he is moving very quickly through a long, dark tunnel. After that he suddenly finds himself at a distance from his body and can now see it with the people around it from outside or alone. He begins to get accustomed to this odd situation and discovers that he possesses a "body" — very different from the physical body left behind — with new properties and powers. Eventually further happenings take place: "Others come to meet and to help him. He glimpses the spirits of relatives and friends who have already died, and a loving, warm spirit of a kind he has never encountered before — a being of light — appears before him. This being asks him a question, nonverbally, to make him evaluate his life and helps him along by showing him a panoramic, instantaneous playback of the major events of his life. At some point he finds himself approaching some sort of barrier or border, apparently representing the limit between earthly life and the next life. Yet he finds that he must go back to the earth, that the time for his death has not yet come. At this point he resists, for by now he is taken up with his experiences in the afterlife and does not want to return. He is overwhelmed by intense feelings of joy, love and peace. Despite his attitude, though, he somehow reunites with his physical body and lives.''[7] That is the "model" — not fully realized in every case — of the process of dying, as described by Moody.[8]

Possible Explanations

The reality of these experiences can neither be disputed nor ignored. There is too much evidence available for us to categorize them as a lot of imaginative lies. But it is quite valid to ask, What do these experiences prove? For Moody, Kübler-Ross, and others they definitely point to the existence of an afterlife, a life which certain people have glimpsed but not fully attained. Hans Küng would disagree. He quotes the work of Ronald K. Siegel of the University of California, psychologist and specialist in psychopharmacy and hallucinations, who claims that there are striking similarities between these accounts and drug-induced hallucinations. He goes on to comment,

> In the extreme situation of the onset of death a psychological protective circuit of the brain prevents the dying person from perceiving the danger of his condition, so that consciousness can escape into a dreamland. Agitations of the central nervous system produce euphoric feelings, extraordinary light stimuli, both simple and complex visions in feverish intensity and rapidity. The overloaded central nervous system simply switches off certain parts of the brain, interposing a kind of shutter between the internal and the external world and allow-

ing the dying person to drift into a sphere without space and time, past and future. At the same time the highly active brain of the dying person produces "internally," unceasingly and unimpeded, pictures from past and future and brings them as far as possible into a meaningful series with the aid of information about death accumulated and perceived as important in the course of life. All this means that experiences close to death should be understood as a kind of final "substitute breathing" of the dying brain, what is known as the last flickering of the fire before it finally dies out . . . . [9]

Küng is not denying the reality of the experience, nor that there may very well be an afterlife. He simply wants it understood that these experiences do not provide adequate proof.

He develops his argument further by making the distinction between clinical and biological death. Clinical death is defined as "that state in which suspension of breathing, of heart activity and brain reaction has been observed, but in which resuscitation — especially by heart massage or artificial respiration — is not completely excluded."[10] By biological death he means "that state in which at least the brain . . . has irrevocably lost its function and can no longer be reanimated. This biological death is certainly definitive: the irreversible loss of vital functions and decay of all organs and tissue."[11] This being the case (and even Moody admits to this) none of the persons who have had such experiences ever *really died*. They were simply going through the final stage of dying and had not, in fact, reached death. Hence Küng would argue that the experience proves nothing about the possibility of life after death. He says, "It is a question here of the last five minutes *before* death and not of an eternal life *after* death."[12] All this would seem to indicate that these phenomena could very well be considered as "this life" experiences, and not experiences of the "next life."

While these experiences do not prove the existence of a life after death, the distinction between clinical and biological death does not rule out the possibility that such experiences could be glimpses into the beyond. It certainly does not prove that they were some kind of hallucination or purely subjective phenomena. The absence of proof on the one side also implies absence of proof on the other. Küng would possibly agree.

The question still remains as to whether we can ascribe any kind of validity to these experiences, and this applies to any of the phenomena we are considering in this chapter. There are empirically minded people who would dismiss any experience that cannot be validated by facts or expressed in such a way that others can share the information. Such mystical experiences are very quickly swept away by such persons as the philosopher A.J. Ayer. He writes, ''We do not deny *a priori* that the mystic is able to discover truths by his own special methods. We wait to hear what are the propositions which embody his discoveries, in order to see whether they are verified or confuted by our own empirical observations . . . . The fact that he cannot reveal what he 'knows,' or even himself devise an empirical test to validate his 'knowledge,' shows that his state of intuition is not a genuinely cognitive state. So that in describing his vision the mystic does not give any information about the external world: he merely gives us indirect information about the condition of his own mind.''[13]

There are other philosophers who are not so definite in their assessment of such experiences. C.D. Broad expresses a more cautious view. ''I am prepared to admit that such experiences occur among people of different races and social traditions and that they have occurred at all periods of history. I am prepared to admit that, although the experiences have differed considerably at different times and places and although the interpretations of them have differed still more, there are probably certain characteristics which are common to them all and suffice to distinguish them from all other kinds of experience. In view of this I think it more likely than not that in religious and mystical experience men come into contact with some Reality or aspect of Reality which they do not come into contact with in any other way.''[14]

This other Reality, referred to by Broad, is sometimes couched in terms which are hard to understand and would invariably be considered as nonsense by someone like Ayer. A typical example of this mystical language is offered by Arthur Koestler as he describes a personal experience when he was in confinement under sentence of death. He felt that his self seemed to drift into another realm. He ends his description in this way: ''Then I was floating . . . in a river of peace . . . . It came from nowhere and went nowhere . . . . Then there was no river and no 'I.' The 'I' had ceased to exist . . . . The 'I' ceases to exist because it has by a kind of mental osmosis established communication with and been dissolved in the universal pool. It is this process of dissolution and limitless expansion which is sensed as the 'oceanic feeling,' as the draining of all tension, the absolute catharsis, the peace that passeth all understanding."[15] One can sense in these words a painful struggle to describe a reality for which the language of our present condition is so woefully inadequate.

We certainly do not have the tools at our disposal to validate or invalidate these phenomena. In a strictly scientific sense we will never be able to prove that there is another life after death. But it is equally true that modern scientific knowledge cannot provide adequate evidence against it. There is sufficient evidence available that we can reasonably explore the possibility of survival, and also study the evidence in a way that need not be considered unscientific. It would be highly prejudicial if we dismissed the evidence out of hand. We do not have to search very far to find examples of how inventors of new knowledge have been quickly ignored or condemned by their contemporaries — and all in the name of good scientific method.

It is reasonable to assume that there are realities we do not yet know about, and realities about which we have only skimmed the surface. The question we ought to be asking is whether these experiences of other possible realities have any value for people as they continue along their spiritual journeys. And in order to examine this more closely we need to look at similar experiences which have been recorded in other writings, notably the Scriptures.

Biblical Examples of Similar Experiences

There is the story of Jacob's dream. "He dreamt that he saw a ladder, which rested on the ground with its top reaching to heaven, and angels of God were going up and down upon it. The Lord was standing beside him and said, 'I am the Lord, the God of your father Abraham and the God of Isaac. This land on which you are lying I will give to you and your descendents. They shall be countless as the dust upon the earth, and you shall spread far and wide, to north and south, to east and west. All the families of the earth shall pray to be blessed as you and your descendents are blessed. I will be with you and I will protect you wherever you go and will bring you back to this land, for I will not leave you until I have done all that I have promised.' Jacob woke from his sleep and said, 'Truly the Lord is in this place, and I did not know it.' Then he was afraid and said, 'How fearsome is this place! This is no other than the house of God, this is the gate of heaven' '' (Genesis 28:12–18). This was a vision which assured Jacob of his place within the purposes of God, and gave him the hope that the God of his forefathers would continue to work through him. He was assured that there was a link between this world and the next.

When the prophet Elijah was threatened with death he fled to the wilderness. In a moment of despair he even asked the Lord to take his life. As he pondered the uselessness of his life, the Lord approached him. It is described in this way: ''A great and strong wind came rending mountains and shattering rocks before him, but the Lord was not in the wind; and after the wind there was an earthquake, but the Lord was not in the earthquake; and after the earthquake fire, but the Lord was not in the fire; and after the fire a low murmuring sound'' (1 Kings 19:11–12). And then Elijah gets the direction he needs. He is promised that his voice will be heard and that he will succeed in his ministry.

A similar vision was experienced by the prophet Isaiah. He was in the temple when he saw the Lord seated upon a throne, high and exalted, and ''about him were attendant seraphim, and each had six wings; one pair covered his face and one pair his feet, and one pair was spread in flight. They were calling ceaselessly to one another, Holy, Holy, Holy is the Lord of Hosts: the whole earth is full of his glory. And, as each one called, the threshold shook to its foundation, while the house was filled with smoke. Then I cried, Woe is me! I am lost, for I am a man of unclean lips and I dwell among a people of unclean lips; yet with these eyes I have seen the King, the Lord of Hosts. Then one of the seraphim flew to me carrying in this hand a glowing coal which he had taken from the altar with a pair of tongs. He touched my mouth with it and said, See, this has touched your lips; your iniquity is removed, and your sin is wiped away. Then I heard the Lord saying, Whom shall I send? Who will go for me? And I answered, Here am I; send me'' (Isaiah 6:1–8).

Again we are given a very imaginative account of another reality, and as a result of this experience Isaiah realizes his call as a prophet. It is interesting to note that in all these accounts the glimpse into the beyond seems to happen when the individual is in a crisis situation and searching for direction.

Probably the most familiar instance of such phenomena is the conversion of St. Paul. As he recounts the event: "I was on the road and nearing Damascus, when suddenly about midday a great light flashed from the sky all around me, and I fell to the ground. Then I heard a voice saying to me, 'Saul, Saul, why do you persecute me?' I answered, 'Tell me, Lord, who you are?' 'I am Jesus of Nazareth,' he said, 'whom you are persecuting.' My companions saw the light, but did not hear the voice that spoke to me. 'What shall I do, Lord?' I said, and the Lord replied, 'Get up and continue your journey to Damascus; there you will be told of all the tasks that are laid upon you.' As I had been blinded by the brilliance of that light, my companions led me by the hand, and so I came to Damascus" (Acts 22:6–11). The reference to a great light is particularly interesting since that kind of experience figures so prominently in other accounts. And here again, it would appear that the rationale for this experience is to enable Paul to find direction in his life.

In one of his letters Paul gives an account of a person who had, what we might call today, an out-of-the-body experience, and from the way he describes the event it is easy to conjecture that it was an experience which Paul had himself. "I know a Christian man who fourteen years ago (whether in the body or out of it, I do not know — God knows) was caught up as far as the third heaven. And I know that this same man (whether in the body or out of it, I do not know — God knows) was caught up into paradise, and heard words so secret that human lips may not repeat them. About such a man as that I am ready to boast; but I will not boast on my own account, except of my weaknesses. If I should choose to boast, it would not be the boast of a fool, for I should be speaking the truth. But I refrain, because I should not like anyone to form an estimate of me which goes beyond the evidence of his own eyes and ears. And so, to keep me from being unduly elated by the magnificence of such revelations, I was given a sharp physical pain which came as Satan's message to bruise me; this was to save me from being unduly elated" (2

Corinthians 12:2–7). Paul is obviously trying to maintain an air of modesty lest he be accused of boasting and displaying a somewhat self-righteous attitude. At the same time he does allude to magnificent revelations which he has had, and in that way subtly suggests to his readers that he does have credibility as a spokesman for the Lord. Paul continually had problems establishing his authority.

If Paul did indeed have these experiences, why does he appear so confused as to whether he was in his body or out of it? This does not seem surprising when we consider accounts of a similar nature. In a number of instances people are able to see their physical body while being aware of a second bodily form. There is the physical body, which the person no longer wants, and the new body which cannot be adequately described. In a sense this ties in with another reference by St. Paul to the existence of a physical body and a spiritual body. Paul does not talk about the next life in terms of a soul being united with God, but rather as a spirit being given some sort of bodily form, which he admits cannot be adequately described (1 Corinthians 15:35–44). This is an admission which is echoed over and over again by those who have experienced this spiritual phenomenon. It is as if people have moved into another reality, a reality which defies description in our three-dimensional language.

Another well-known account which is full of mystical imagery is the Book of Revelation. Just to quote one of many visionary experiences, the writer describes his vision of heaven. "Then I saw a new heaven and a new earth, for the first heaven and the first earth had vanished, and there was no longer any sea. I saw the holy city, new Jerusalem, coming down out of heaven from God, made ready like a bride adorned for her husband. I heard a loud voice proclaiming from the throne: 'Now at last God has his dwelling among men! He will dwell among them and they shall be his people, and God himself will be with them' " (Revelation 21:1–3). It could be argued that this book consists of nothing more than codified imagery, expressing hopeful expectations in a way which only a Christian reader would understand. It may, in other words, simply be a piece of descriptive writing and not an account of an actual mystical experience. Since we will never know the answer to that question, we can only assume that at least the writer believed mysticism to be a valid vehicle for conveying the truth, and that he would no doubt consider such experiences as acceptable gifts of God's grace.

The other pieces of scriptural evidence which need to be considered are the appearances of Jesus immediately after his death. There are some unusual characteristics in these stories which relate to the subject at hand. The first account is the appearance to Mary outside the tomb. She had come there to prepare the body for burial but found the tomb empty. While she laments the loss of the body, Jesus appears. She thinks it is the gardener and actually addresses him: "If it is you, sir, who removed him, tell me where you have laid him, and I will take him away" (John 20:15). It is only when he pronounces her name, no doubt in a way that would be familiar to her, that she recognizes him.

On another occasion two disciples were on the road to Emmaus. Jesus appears and talks to them for the whole day. They invite him to stay and dine with them. And it is only in the breaking of the bread that they recognize him (Luke 24:13–35). Similarly when Jesus appeared to the disciples following this incident they thought that they were seeing a ghost. Jesus had to show his hands and feet in order to convince them who he was (Luke 24:36–43). Later Jesus appeared to them while they were fishing and talked to them. We are told that they did not know it was the Lord. Only after they had caught a multitude of fish did they recognize him.

It is possible to explain this lack of recognition in terms of emotional disbelief. But this is not entirely satisfactory. The frequency of these mistaken apearances, and to the same people on different occasions, seems to indicate that some change had taken place, and that new methods of recognition had to be adopted. He was known in the pronouncement of a name, in the breaking the bread, in the symbols of his death, and in a miraculous catch of fish.

But just how much can we glean from these accounts, without indulging in expository preaching, is a moot point. They really only hint at the possibility that there may be a transitional state immediately after death where some kind of bodily existence is experienced, even though changed in some way. It is interesting that when Mary rushed up to Jesus he responded: "Do not cling to me, for I have not yet ascended to the Father" (John 20:17). It would seem that what had happened to Jesus was not yet complete. But again, this is only a hint that those who have had some glimpse into the beyond or a "life after death" experience may have broached this transitional state. In so many instances people have said that during such an experience they felt that they were moving towards something, but that they never quite reached their goal. The sense of finality or completion was not there. It is also interesting to note that those who have experienced these phenomena report that the methods of recognizing people were different. They just knew, in some strange way, whom they were meeting, but it was unlike the way we recognize people in this life.

None of this proves the existence of a life after death. Nor can these events in Scripture prove the validity of the experiences we are considering. They can only serve as further pieces of evidence, pointing to the possibility of other realities we have yet to understand.

Our Response to the Experiences

But the question still remains, What is the appropriate pastoral response to these experiences? Since their origin cannot be proven in any conclusive way, are we simply to accept them blindly, or can we test the value of these experiences within the life of the recipient?

Perhaps the first appropriate response would be to set the experience against one's theological background. How does the experience compare with one's understanding of God, of the way God communicates with humanity, and of the promise of a resurrected life. For example, the resurrection of Jesus can be interpreted as God's way of indicating to us that the next life will be one in which we will enjoy community. Just as the physical body now is the means whereby we can communicate and relate to each other, so in the next life we will be given a form whereby we can continue to live in community with others. We will not disappear into the Godhead like a drop of water falling into the ocean. We will maintain our individuality and identity. We are also promised that this community will be filled with intense love and compassion. Needless to say, we accept all this in faith based on the life and teaching of Jesus. But it is interesting that the character of some of these mystical experiences appears to be consistent with what has been promised to us in Scripture. In the accounts of life-after-death experiences, people may recall meeting others who meant a great deal to them. They felt an intense love around them. They were able to recognize others and had a sense of personal identity. In both the life-after-death experiences and the out-of-body experiences, people remember feeling a sense of wholeness. These elements within the experience seem quite consistent with what has been described in Scripture as the resurrected life, and this can have the effect of reinforcing one's belief and understanding of what God has promised for us. In this sense the experience can prove to be of value for the recipient.

The experience of having a life review or the feeling that a whole lifetime has passed in front of one is possibly an excellent way of describing judgement. The image of God as a divine magistrate dispensing blessings and curses is not particularly appropriate. While there may very well be a reckoning, it is one which we will possibly do *for ourselves*. God will not have to say a word, we will just *know* within ourselves the value of our past life.

The poetic imagery sometimes used to describe what people have seen and heard in these experiences may suggest that the next life is just an infinite improvement on this life. The imagery is obviously not to be taken literally. At the same time it is not inconceivable or completely unacceptable that people should receive such images. In most cases there is the experience of moving towards something else. The final goal has not been reached. As Hans Küng reminds us, these people are not dead but are going through the last stages of dying. If the images mean anything, they are possibly symbolic of all those things in this life which stand for beauty, love, and peace. In many of the accounts, the content of the experience reflects what the person has valued within his or her own religion and culture. The images used are the only means that person has of describing an existence which is intensely good and beautiful, but they cannot indicate the precise nature of the next life. This was expressed rather candidly by a former patient at St. Christopher's Hospice in a poem composed just days before he died.

The imagination runs riot
In visualizing heaven.
Is heaven really

Like the background music
To a Hollywood biblical epic?
Is heaven a magnified
Hallelujah Chorus
Sung by an augmented
Huddersfield Choir?
We can easily imagine
What heaven is not.
All I need know
This side of the trumpets sounding
Is that heaven
Is the vision of my God
Seeing all things and acting in Him.[16]

Sidney G. Reeman

Another appropriate pastoral response is to ask what effect the experience has had on the individual? It may have been an interesting and enjoyable event, but has it produced anything meaningful for that person's life? In some cases it seems that people become far more aware of what is truly valuable in life. Relationships become more meaningful and people discover a lot about themselves which can lead to personal growth. When these results are evident, it is a sign that the experience has been of value, and gives us good reason to trust in the event. But this does not necessarily mean that every experience, be it a dream, a vision, an out-of-body experience, or a life-after-death experience, will be a pleasant event. The experience could be frightening and lead to a great deal of anxiety. It could be that the experience is a reminder of some unfinished business, a reconciliation that needs to be made, or a suppressed guilt that has risen to the surface. But the experience can still be of value to the recipient if appropriate steps are taken to deal with the significance and meaning of the event. Any experience, be it pleasant or unpleasant, can lead to personal growth.

Dreams and Premonitions

The kind of experiences which seem to occur more frequently in the final stages of dying are dreams and premonitions. Dying patients may indicate that dreams convey messages and have deep spiritual significance. Unfortunately some caregivers have difficulty responding to dream experiences and simply discount them as the meaningless ramblings of a deteriorating mind. But the reluctance to take them seriously may be due to a feeling of awkwardness and an inability to interpret them. Some caregivers may feel that they are expected to explain the event and derive some meaning from it. But this is not necessarily what the patient wants. A far better approach is to encourage the patient to discover for himself or herself what value there might be in the experience.

The premonition of death is not unlike the dream. It reflects an inner realization that death is approaching. (Derek Doyle estimates that 80 to 90 per cent of dying patients know intuitively that their life is coming to an end.[1]) In some cases these premonitons bring a degree of anxiety, but in the majority of instances there is a sense of peace and acceptance. Again, the appropriate response is to help the patient discover the value of the experience.

Visions and Visitations

Another common phenomenon is the vision or visitation. This may happen either to patients in the dying process or to families after the death has occurred. The recipient may feel hesitant to speak about such an experience for fear of being labelled psychotic. Hence, it is important not to give the impression that the reality or the unreality of the experience is being pre-judged. The content of the message may vary. It can come in the form of a word of advice, or just a quiet reassurance that all is well. Again, such experiences have to be taken seriously with a view to determining what value can be derived from them. An examination of similar experiences in the past, especially in the Old and New Testaments, seems to indicate that they occurred for a specific reason, one which gave direction to an individual or community. Value and purpose were associated with the event.

Caregivers may be loathe to discuss such an experience with a patient, and this is understandable. When you are standing at the foot of the bed and the patient asks you to move over because his departed mother has just appeared, it can be a little disconcerting. But the feeling of awkwardness may be partly due to the caregiver's expectation that the experience *must* be analysed. It could be a wishful projection from the patient's mind or a real happening. It cannot be proven either way. The appropriate response is to help the patient discover what value it might have for his or her condition.

It is true that the church speaks about the communion of saints and that within the family of God we are at one with the departed through our common faith. But the church has never sanctioned the practice of endeavouring to communicate with the dead. There is little record of this practice in Scripture, except in one instance where Saul was so desperate for advice he found someone to call up the spirit of Samuel, and this experience not only distressed Saul, but eventually led to his death (1 Samuel 28:3–20). If there is to be any communication, one must think of it as a gift and not something to be solicited.

The experience of visitations sometimes raises the issue about whether the dead are aware of what is happening to the living. This is one of those speculative questions which cannot lead to any valid or useful answer. It may be that the people who ask such questions are really expressing their grief over the loss of someone very dear to them, and they would like to believe that the relationship is still being maintained in some way. There may also be the fear that the departed will have progressed so far in the next life that the one left behind will not be able to catch up and renew the relationship later. Unfortunately there is no way of knowing the condition of those relationships in the next life. It may be comforting to reflect on the belief that at some point loved ones will be joined together again, but the nature of that relationship could be significantly different from what is experienced in this life.

There are certainly no easy explanations. But the fact remains that these experiences do occur, and it is incumbent upon caregivers to respond appropriately. It may be that these phenomena are more frequent than we realize, and by addressing them seriously, patients may feel less reticent about sharing them with us. Whatever they mean, they are real to the recipient and need to be acknowledged by those who are providing spiritual care.

Notes

1 Raymond A. Moody, *Life After Life* (New York: Bantam Books, 1975); Karlis Osis and Erlendur Haraldsson, *At the Hour of Death* (New York: Avon Books, 1977); Elisabeth Kübler-Ross, *On Children and Death* (New York: Macmillan Publishing Company, 1983).

2 Rosalind Heywood, "Attitudes to death in the light of dreams and other out-of-the-body experience," *Man's Concern with Death* (London: Hodder and Stoughton, 1968), p. 199.

3 Enneads IV, viii, 1, McKenna's translation, quoted from Rosalind Heywood, *op. cit.*, p. 203.

4 Rosalind Heywood, *op. cit.*, p. 197.

5 *Ibid.*, p. 197–198.

6 Raymond Moody, *op. cit.*, p. 35.

7 *Ibid.*, p. 22.

8 Hans Küng, *Eternal Life?* (New York: Doubleday and Company, Inc., 1984), p. 10.

9 *Ibid.*, p. 17.

10 *Ibid.*, p. 19.

11 *Ibid.*, p. 19.

12 *Ibid.*, p. 20.

13 A.J. Ayer, *Language, Truth and Logic* (Gollancz, 1936), p. 118–119.

14 C.D. Broad, *Religion, Philosophy, and Psychical Research* (Routledge and Kegan Paul, 1953), p. 172–173.

15 Arthur Koestler, *The Invisible Writing* (Hamish Hamilton, Collins, 1954), p. 352–353.

16 Cicely Saunders, ed., *Beyond All Pain* (London: S.P.C.K., 1983), p. 62.

17 Derek Doyle, ed., *Palliative Care, The Management of Far-Advanced Illness* (London: Croom Helm, 1984), p. 474.

Practising Pastoral Care

Certain words carry connotations which sometimes unjustly limit their meaning. This is especially true for the words *pastoral care*. If you were to walk into a hospital and ask for the pastoral-care department, you would inevitably be introduced to the chaplain or some theologically trained person. You would undoubtedly be surprised if you came face to face with a gynaecologist. Pastoral work has become a speciality like all the other departments in our health-care system.

But pastoral work can become self-limiting if it is done *only* by the official pastoral caregivers. It may, indeed, be a speciality, but it is a speciality which can be shared in varying degrees by anyone associated with caring for the sick. Many doctors, nurses, and family members are, in fact, often engaged in pastoral care. It is tempting to think that, unless one is being visited by a "religious" person, or is engaged in "religious" conversation, pastoral care is not being practised. But just as spirituality should not be confused with "religiosity," pastoral care should not be confused with "professional pastors."

If a patient asks any caregiver to act as a spiritual confidant, that request should be honoured. The chosen caregiver may want to consult with a professional pastoral-care worker when issues arise which are difficult to understand or contend with, but it is most important that the choice of the patient be respected at all times.

One might assume that pastoral care will be requested only by people with a strong religious faith, but this is to seriously limit the scope of pastoral care. Anyone who is engaged in the search for life's meaning will appreciate pastoral help. The word *pastoral* has strong associations with the concept of shepherding. And it is the work of a shepherd gently to guide people in their spiritual journeys, not to drag them through a prescribed route. Since everyone is engaged in some kind of journey, the compassionate presence of a pastoral caregiver will always be appreciated.

Unfortunately, even patients themselves may have a limited notion of pastoral care. On many occasions people have initially responded to my pastoral visit with the apologetic comment, "Well, I haven't been a very good churchgoer," as if they do not deserve my intervention because of a poor batting average with the institution. In most instances this notion can quietly be laid to rest during subsequent visits, but it possibly accounts for the hesitation on the part of many people to request a pastoral visit. They feel that they have not earned the right to receive such services.

In the course of a pastoral intervention one will often sense the absence of denominational or religious barriers. During the course of life we put great stock in ecclesiastical differences, but at the end of life they seem to lose their importance. Even people of different religious faiths can discover meaningful common ground, and engage in a dialogue which both parties find acceptable. Death seems to have a levelling influence and helps people focus on what is fundamental and basic to human life. We think of ourselves not as Presbyterians, Anglicans, Roman Catholics, Jews, or Muslims, but rather as children of God.

The Role of the Chaplain

While anyone may be called upon to provide pastoral care, it is important that we consider the role of the chaplain. Can we define the chaplain's duties in such a way that he or she will occupy a specific place in the team of health-care professionals? We need to examine how the chaplain's role has been conceived in the past and how the contemporary chaplain functions today.

In recent years the role of the chaplain has changed considerably. The Rev. John Swift, director of Pastoral Care at the Institute of Pastoral Studies in Ottawa, describes the change in this way. "The certified chaplain is well prepared to function in health care settings with skill and knowledge: he is a specialist in ministry. The stereotyped chaplain — a doddering old cleric, unable to handle a parish, who wanders from room to room praying and reading the Bible at patients and dispensing communion wafers ad infinitum — is being replaced by a competent professional."[1]

John Swift has caricatured the role of the chaplains somewhat bluntly, but we need not assume that he is underestimating the significance of Bible reading or the sacraments. I would interpret his comments to indicate that the present-day chaplain has now increased his professional competence beyond those duties practised in the past.

But if the chaplain is now a "competent professional," wherein lies his competence? Today there is a far greater concern for clinical training in the preparation for chaplaincy work, and this certainly helps the chaplain acquire a more proficient expertise in counselling techniques. But this has led some people to suspect that chaplains are becoming psychologists in ecclesiastical clothing. Joseph Fichter observes, "Psychologist Bernard Spilka and his associates find that there is a trend towards secularism among the clergy, a rejection of traditional and spiritual roles and a preference for the role of comforter and counselor. Their research shows the minister often neglecting whatever competence they had in religious knowledge and in pastoral theology and simply imitating the language and concepts of clinical psychology."[2] There is an obvious danger here for chaplains to rely on concepts which can be analysed, measured, and quantified in order to escape from problematic religious concepts which do not have easy answers. This is not in any way to underestimate the importance of clinical knowledge, but total reliance on this knowledge does not provide the chaplain with any kind of unique role.

Andrew D. Elia uses a number of phrases to describe the role and qualifications of a chaplain. He says such a person "requires all the psychology, philosophy and faith that he can muster." He must be a "genial, well-adjusted person" and "a leader of men." He must be attuned to the "dynamics of human personality" and have "adequate clinical training."[3] While these may be excellent qualifications, they seem equally appropriate for a psychologist.

In a somewhat different vein, John Swift summarizes the role of the chaplain: "The chaplain meets people in both relational and cognative ways . . . . The chaplain's principal tool is his own being and his willingness to communicate deeply with others . . . . The chaplain can give informed and discriminating professional opinions on ethical/moral decisions and on particular concerns . . . . The chaplain is a member of the interdisciplinary health care team . . . . The chaplain can minister to other members of the team."[4] These excerpts could obviously be expanded and may not adequately represent Swift's excellent article on this subject, but they do help us focus on what might be considered as the unique nature of the chaplain's role.

Above all, chaplains present themselves as representatives of God and of a particular belief system. Two words which occur most frequently in the descriptions of chaplaincy roles are *symbolic* and *representative*. Just as the doctor represents a body of medical knowledge, so the chaplain represents a body of spiritual knowledge which is designed to provide direction in life. He or she stands as a symbol of a caring community, people who are committed to serving others in a loving and prayerful manner. But underlying all this symbolic language is the one basic theme — the chaplain is the representative of God. Unfortunately this can raise some serious problems.

The response of the patient to the chaplain will, to a large extent, be conditioned by his or her image of God. One of the prevailing images (and this is typical in a variety of religious faiths) is that of a judgemental figure. God is the divine magistrate in the sky, taking careful account of man's actions and words with a view to pronouncing sentence on judgement day. This is a predominant theme in both the Old and New Testaments. It has been instilled in us through our catechetical instruction, it permeates our traditional liturgies, and it has possibly caused considerable guilt and fear in the minds of religious people.

This imagery is reinforced by the value system which chaplains represent. They are seen as "holy" persons and stand for a way of life which can quickly mirror the "unholiness" in the patient. The presence of the chaplain can also have the effect of reminding the patient of previous doubts about the faith which have accumulated over the years. And this, in turn, can lead to a degree of anxiety, especially when combined with a belief in a righteous and judgemental God.

While it is important for a person to make peace with God, it is imperative that the chaplain convey such a compassionate presence that the person will modify his or her image of the creator and begin to believe that forgiveness and reconciliation are really achievable goals. The chaplain can also be an effective agent in helping the patient realize what has been of value in life and so engage in a search for meaning. In a very real sense the chaplain stands before the patient as one who is most willing to engage in this search.

One of the complaints expressed by chaplains is that they are often bypassed by patients and families alike when it comes to discussing spiritual matters, or for that matter any issue of major importance. In an interesting survey done in twelve areas of England and Wales involving 960 cases, the question was asked of general practitioners and district nurses, Who should be involved in telling a dying patient about his or her prognosis? Eighty-nine per cent of the general practitioners voted for the doctor, and 11 per cent for the chaplain or parish priest; 79 per cent of the nurses favoured the doctor and 15 per cent the priest.[5] The conclusion was drawn that either the priest had abdicated his role or was not given the opportunity to engage in this role. While it would seem reasonable to expect the doctor to provide the initial information about the diagnosis, it is unfortunate that the chaplain was not commonly understood to share in this information-giving process. His or her potential to contribute is often overlooked.

Sometimes it is possible to rectify this situation by contracting with a doctor to indicate when he or she intends to speak to the patient, so that the pastoral caregiver can be on the scene immediately to provide additional support. But this only happens when doctor and chaplain share a mutual respect for each other's professional capabilities. If this is missing, then the chaplain's contribution may not be sought.

But why does the chaplain get bypassed? In some instances there may be little confidence in the capabilities of the pastoral caregiver. Sometimes this lack of confidence is justified. But the main reason for the breakdown in communication may simply be a matter of accessibility. And this applies not only to local parish clergy but also to resident chaplains in a hospital. Chaplains have to cover so much ground that there is insufficient opportunity to spend adequate time with each individual. Since spiritual matters do not arise at prescribed times in the day when the chaplain just happens to be around, the patient may select someone more immediately available. And since it would be most inappropriate for the chaplain to intervene when a choice has been made by the patient, the role of the chaplain changes to becoming that of a supportive team member to the person who has been chosen.

There is another dimension to the chaplain's role which is sometimes overlooked. This has to do with the representative function of the chaplain. The presence of the chaplain can have the effect of evoking within the patient a concern to deal with spiritual matters. In the words of Derek Doyle, the visit of the chaplain "can also have the effect of provoking the patient into exploring some of the more profound issues integral to a serious illness."[6] The same idea was expressed by Phyllis Smyth, chaplain at the Royal Victoria Hospital in Montreal. She said, "You become in the eyes of the patient a representative of whatever the spiritual dimension of life is," and in that capacity "it is like a key in the door." It may very well be that the patient will eventually choose someone else to see what lies behind the door, but the chaplain has been the person who has enabled the door to be opened.

Elizabeth Dingwall, who is the palliative care nurse at the Palliative Care Centre in the Halifax Infirmary, recently commented that it was not a disadvantage that the chaplain's role cannot be clearly defined. She felt that the chaplain was freer than members of other disciplines and was not so closely locked into one particular position. She felt that this "fuzzy role" was an advantage, and gave the chaplain the opportunity to be a "cohesive catalyst" both with patients and staff members. We are often prone to define roles for the sake of security, and so establish our own private piece of turf which will give us a sense of professional well-being. If we are supposed to function as an interdisciplinary team, there have to be points where disciplines overlap and somehow join forces in the total care of the patient. We all know that within the health-care system there is a constant concern to review and update job descriptions. In principle this is a good thing, but it can also be taken to the extreme, and we can find caregivers becoming jealous of their particular role. It would be sad if chaplains fell prey to this temptation. Maybe this "fuzzy role" can also suggest the need for members of all disciplines to be conscious of their interrelation, and so provide better assurance for the total care of the patient.

The Place of Prayer in Spiritual Care

One of the predominant roles of religious leaders throughout the centuries, and in every religion, is that of an intermediary between the people and God. These leaders stand before God as the representatives of the people, and also before the people as the representatives of God. All kinds of ceremonies have been devised from the most simple to the most elaborate, but in every ritual a person is usually set apart to express the hopes, the needs, and the praises of the people of God. Prayer becomes the medium of communication with God.

Even though religious leaders are intimately associated with the life of prayer, it is not their exclusive right. Just as anyone may be chosen to be a spiritual confidant, so anyone may be asked to engage in prayer. Some doctors and nurses have occasionally been surprised when a patient has asked them to say a prayer. Their first reaction is to call for the chaplain. But this is to abdicate the trust which the patient has just offered, and can give the impression that the patient has been wrong in choosing them as spiritual confidants. To engage in prayer is a very sacred act, but not as onerous as one may think. But what is the purpose of prayer?

The ultimate purpose of prayer is to recognize, either verbally or silently, that we are in the presence of God. It is the conscious effort to communicate with God in such a way that we reveal what is truly on our minds, and perhaps become aware of what is on God's mind. It is an activity which brings out the best and the worst in a person because the person who prays knows only too well that God cannot be fooled. Prayer is a great leveller and brings a person to a degree of honesty and openness which we seldom achieve in our normal relations in life. But prayer is more than just a vertical relationship with God. It can also create and enrich a horizontal relationship with other people. Harold Kushner makes the same point. ''Prayer, when it is offered in the right way, redeems people from isolation. It assures them that they need not feel alone and abandoned. It lets them know that they are part of a greater reality, with more depth, more hope, more courage, and more of a future than any individual could have by himself.''[7]

This is borne out by the experiences of the patients in St. Christopher's Hospice. Enid Henke had lived a very active life and found dependence very hard to bear. She finally discovered peace, and it was largely through the prayers of other people. She dictated her thoughts during the month before she died.

A friend and I were considering life and its purpose. I said, even with increasing paralysis and loss of speech, I believed there was a purpose for my life, but I was not sure what it was at that particular time. We agreed to pray about it for a week. I was then sure that my present purpose is simply to receive other person's prayers and kindness and to link together all those who are lovingly concerned about me, many of whom are unknown to one another. After a while my friend said: ''It must be hard to be a wounded Jew when, by nature, you would rather be the Good Samaritan.''

It is hard: it would be unbearable were it not for my belief that the wounded man and the Samaritan are inseparable. It was the helplessness of the one that brought out the best in the other and linked them together.

In reflecting on the parable, I am particularly interested in the fact that we are not told the wounded man recovered. I have always assumed that he did, but now it occurs to me that even if he did not recover, the story will stand as a perfect example of true neighbourliness. You will remember that the story concludes with the Samaritan asking the innkeeper to take care of the man, but he assures him of his own continuing interest and support: so, the innkeeper becomes linked.

If, as my friend suggested, I am cast in the role of the wounded man, I am not unmindful of the modern day counterparts of the Priest and the Levite, but I am overwhelmed by the kindness of so many ''Samaritans.'' There are those who, like you, have been praying for me for a long time and constantly reassure me of continued interest and support. There are many others who have come into my life — people I would never have met had I not been in need, who are now being asked to take care of me. I like to think that all of us have been linked together for a purpose which will prove a means of blessing to us all.[8]

This is clearly a case where prayer has not only linked people in an open and trusting relationship, but also has given meaning to someone who felt helpless and dependent. It is this discovery of meaning that represents one of the objects of spirituality. Prayer can be the medium through which we find purpose for our relationships with each other as well as our relationship with God.

The hesitancy to engage in prayer when faced with a serious illness is largely due to some confusion as to what one should pray about. Are we to pray for a miraculous cure, or would this build up false hopes? Are we to use some general prayer in a devotional manual, or make up something ourselves? Where do we begin when someone asks us to pray with them? The traditional distinction between formal and extemporaneous prayer can become a contentious issue among different denominations. It is pointless to argue which is the superior method. Much will depend on what is meaningful to the patient.

It is most helpful to begin a prayer by focussing on the presence of God. One might call this setting the appropriate atmosphere. Sometimes this is referred to as a "call to worship" which figures prominently in most liturgical circumstances. It is also important to make the prayer as realisitic and specific as possible. One has to try and determine where the patient is in his or her spiritual journey. If there are feelings of loneliness, then we might focus on God's compassionate presence, and how this can be manifested through the lives of loved ones. If there are feelings of guilt, it would be appropriate to provide reassurances of God's forgiveness. If there is a concern about unfinished business, it would be fitting to ask for courage and wisdom to make the right decisions. If people have doubts about their relationship with God, it would be helpful to remind them that God responds to faith even the size of a mustard seed. And when there does not seem to be any clear focus for the prayer, it would be quite appropriate to ask the patient what he or she wants to pray about. The most important thing is that the prayer should be relevant and reach patients where they need the most help at that particular time. But all of this assumes, of course, that time has been spent determining the needs of the patient which then become the content of this communication with God. We must be careful not to be too perfunctory in the delivery of our prayers.

We should not wait too long before we engage in prayer. Far too often clergy end a visit with a prayer, and it seems as if this is just a way of saying goodbye. It is very helpful to spend some time after the prayer, either just being silent with the patient or continuing to reflect on the issues raised by the prayer. Prayer can lead to some important insights, and there should be an opportunity to share them. The practice of holding a person's hand during the prayer can be most effective as long as it does not constitute an invasion of privacy. Touching can communicate a great deal, from you to the patient, in the sense that you really care, and also from the patient to you, because what you are saying is what they need to hear. When the patient's grip tightens at the end of the prayer, it can convey the message, "Thank you. Stay a little longer. I have something important going on inside of me, and I want to share it with you, even in silence."

We would do well to keep the prayer short and to the point. It is better to have short prayers more frequently than long prayers only occasionally. Cicely Saunders has said that no book or card of prayers that she has ever seen has been simple or short enough.[9] We must remember that the attention span of some patients can be very limited.

It is worth commenting at this point about saying prayers with patients who appear to be comatose and not able to respond either verbally or by any movement of the hand or eyes. We know that hearing is the last sense to fail, and for this reason spoken prayer is appropriate. It is good to reassure the patient that we know they can hear what is being said. If the patient can hear but cannot respond, the sense of frustration must be extreme and our reassurances can have a very calming effect. If, on the other hand, the patient cannot hear what is being said, nothing has been lost. Besides all this, we should never think that prayers are only relevant for those who are conscious. If we are prepared to pray for someone who is not in our midst, we can certainly pray for someone who is comatose.

In some hospices and palliative care units the practice of saying a prayer with the family immediately after the death of a loved one has helped the family accept the reality of the death. At the Royal Victoria Hospital in Montreal the team members who are present gather with the family to read the following prayer:

> Our God, in whose presence we came into life, in whose care we live and die, we come at this moment of death to remember with one another the life of _____ who has lived with us. Our love goes with him/her as we now, in silence, commend him/her to your care.[10]

This is similar to the prayer which I frequently use prior to the commital at the graveside but which could also be said immediately following death.

> For the assurance and hope of our faith, and for the saints whom you have received into you eternal joy, we thank you, Heavenly Father. And especially now we lift up our hearts in gratitude for the life of _____, our brother/sister now gone from among us; for all your goodness to him/her; for all that he/she was to those who loved him/her; and for everything in his/her life which reflected your goodness and your love. Let us thank God for _____ life, each of us recalling what he/she has meant to us. (Followed by a short period of silence.) We now commend him/her to God's sure keeping.

At St. Christopher's Hospice the following non-sectarian prayers have been found to be appropriate.

> Unto Thee, O Lord, we commend the soul of Thy servant, that dying unto the world, he may live with Thee; and whatsoever sins he has committed through the frailty of earthly life, we beseech Thee to wipe away by Thy loving and merciful forgiveness.

> Go forth from this world, O Christian soul; in the name of God the Father who created thee; in the name of Jesus who suffered for thee; in the name of the Holy Spirit who strengtheneth thee.

> May thy portion this day be in peace, and thy dwelling in Paradise.

> O Saviour of the world, who by Thy Cross and precious blood hast redeemed us, save us and help us we humbly beseech Thee, O Lord.[11]

There will be times when pastoral caregivers are called upon to administer the Last Rites. While the request may be made with the best of intentions, the terminology can be somewhat misleading. It conjures up the idea that since science has done all it can, the only recourse is to call upon the priest. The Roman Catholic Church has decided to call this liturgy the Sacrament of the Sick, and it is now being used for people other than those who are at the point of death. Nevertheless, there is a very real place for prayer when death is imminent.

A peculiar phenomenon sometimes occurs when prayers are offered at this time, a phenomenon which is difficult to explain. In a number of instances patients have died shortly after the prayers have been offered. It may be that some of these patients were very close to death at the time, but there are also cases where the prognosis has not suggested immediate death, and yet death came very quickly after the ritual. This can make the caregiver feel like the harbinger of death.

One possible explanation is that the prayer gave the person "permission to leave." Our natural instinct is to tenaciously hang on to life, and the will to live sometimes draws out a person's life expectancy, even for those who are comatose. It would seem that some prayers can have the effect of enabling a person to attain a sense of peace with God and so to let go of life. It would, of course, be irresponsible to tell a person it is time to go, and for that reason the words expressed in some services for the dying such as, "Depart, O Christian soul, out of this world" or "May thy rest be this day in peace, and thy dwelling-place in the Paradise of God," are sometimes inappropriate (from *The Book of Common Prayer*, Anglican). It is one thing to say these words over the dead but quite another to read them to the living. It is possible to constuct a prayer which helps people peacefully to place themselves in the hands of God, enables them to identify their will with the will of God, and provides for a peaceful departure.

Rituals before and after Death

In many ways death has become a technical matter reserved for the professionals, be they medical personnel or funeral directors. The family has little or no part in the final preparations either before or after death. Even pastoral caregivers are very often not notified of the patient's condition and have little opportunity to suggest traditional ceremonial rites which might bring comfort to the patient and family. This has resulted in a growing neglect of ritualistic practices.

William Wendt has defined rituals in this way. "Death rituals, by definition, are specific behaviors and activities that enable humans to negotiate the oft-times treacherous corridor that stretches between the moment of separation from the familiar and that of entry into the world of the new, and to be transformed by what takes place in the passage. Such rituals can help people accept the experiences of death — before, during, and after."[12] It is interesting to note how many of our liturgical rites speak of this passage from death to new life. In Baptism a person dies to the old man and becomes a new man in Christ. Holy Communion is a celebration of the death and resurrection of Christ. The service of Confirmation is a conscious declaration that one is ready to die to a dependent relationship within the Christian family and live as an independent responsible member of the church. Marriage involves a kind of death to one set of relationships in order to create a new family. And, of course, funerals are designed to remind us of the passage from death to life.

Such rituals are related to hope, the hope of healing and new life, if not of the body then certainly of the spirit. And two rituals directly related to this idea are the annointing with oil and the laying on of hands. Both these rituals are intensely personal, and through acts of touching, convey and illicit a very personal response. Such actions are important to a person who may be feeling alienated or abandoned. Ritual physical contact is a symbolic declaration of a caring relationship.

There are other ancient rituals such as the watching and washing of the body which might be considered. Rituals such as these can assist the survivors recognize the reality of the death, and allow them the opportunity to show one final act of respect for a loved one. Some kind of ceremony, in which there is family involvement, needs to be introduced at this point. Very often nurses and doctors are seen to dispose of the body in a quick and perfunctory manner, and this is interpreted as insensitivity. But if there is no ceremony available, what else can the medical personnel do? There is no reason why provision of time, space, and community could not be made at this point to assist friends and family in the recognition of the reality facing them and the initiation of the grieving process.

The old custom of the wake served a very useful purpose in allowing friends and family to tell stories and so celebrate the person's life. It was a way of establishing the memory of the departed. Because it took place in the home, it could bring back many happy associations, and in turn allow the grieving process to begin. It has been noted that the laying out of the body in the home is gradually becoming more acceptable in our present day.[13]

It is important to say something about funerals. There is a growing trend today towards the practice of cremation and along with this a tendency to streamline funeral services. The request for a quick private funeral may be motivated by a concern for the next of kin, but minimizing this ritual can have the unfortunate effect of delaying the grieving process. A great deal of care must be taken to ensure that the purpose of the funeral ritual is achieved, because to all intents and purposes this ritual is really for the living, not the departed.

Whatever form the ritual may take, there are certain elements which need to retained. In a few churches the practice of giving a eulogy has virtually been abandoned. Some preachers may use the address as an opportunity to put the "fear of God" into the survivors, which is not a particulary appropriate message for those who come to pay their last respects. Homilies should be designed to provide reassurance and comfort for the bereaved, and they need to be presented tactfully and with brevity. It is very beneficial to inject a personal note into the address. And even if the departed is not well known, a brief conversation with the family will usually reveal a few points about the person's character. The address can then mention the contribution which the person has made during his or her lifetime. In that way it is a celebration of what has given meaning and purpose to the person's life. It becomes a testimony of personal spirituality.

It is not customary for the family to make any comments during the funeral service, but this can be a most helpful addition to the service both from the standpoint of the bereaved and those paying their last respects. I remember a father speaking about his baby girl who had lived only a few months. He assured everyone that he understood how difficult it was for them to find the right words to say, but that this really did not matter. It was simply our presence that provided the support needed at this time. It was a beautiful personal gesture and helped all of us to face the reality of the death. I can remember celebrating the requiem eucharist for my father and taking the opportunity to speak of my love and respect for him. It helped me accept the reality of his death and resolve some of my own personal grief. In every ritual there needs to be some kind of personal element which will help people face the reality of what has happened, and provide them with the opportunity to continue the grieving process.

Far too often our models of pastoral care, either in terms of ceremonies or formalized prayers, convey ideas which may not be relevant to the circumstances at hand. We can very easily fill our rituals with clichés and fail to address the thoughts and feelings going on inside the patient and the members of the family. If there is anger, bitterness, and resentment, it needs to be brought out into the open. If there is fear and doubt, it should not be clouded over with pious phrases that deny the spiritual space of the grieving person. Each moment of crisis during the passage from life to death has a specific character and requires a unique response. It is the job of the pastoral caregiver to identify how a person is coping with the crisis and to construct a pastoral intervention which is both relevant and appropriate.

Notes

1 John K. Swift, "The Chaplain's role in caring for the dying: toward a new understanding," *Canadian Medical Association Journal* 115, (July 17, 1976), p. 181.

2 Joseph H. Fichter, *Religion and Pain* (New York: Crossroad, 1981), p. 110.

3 Andrew D. Elia, "Spiritual needs in the care of the patient," *Pastoral Psychology* (April, 1957), p. 23-24.

4 John K. Swift, *op. cit.*, p. 182 and 185.

5 Ann Cartwright, Lisbeth Hockey, John L. Anderson, *Life Before Death* (London: Routledge and Kegan Paul, 1973), p. 183.

6 Derek Doyle, *Palliative Care: The Management of Far-Advanced Illness* (London: Croom Helm, 1984), p. 416.

7 Harold S. Kushner, *When Bad Things Happen to Good People* (New York: Avon Books, 1981), p. 121.

8 Cicely Saunders, *Beyond All Pain* (London: S.P.C.K., 1983), p. 10.

9 Cicely Saunders, "I was sick and you visited me," *In the Service of Medicine — A Quarterly Paper* 42 (July 1965), p. 2.

10 Brenda Halton, "PCS Experience in meeting spiritual needs," *The*

R.V.H. Manual on Palliative/Hospice Care (New York: Arno Press, 1980), p. 256.

11 Richard Lamerton, "Care of the dying," *Nursing Times* 69 (January 18, 1973), p. 89.

12 William A. Wendt, "Death rituals," *The American Journal of Hospice Care* (1984), p. 25.

13 *Ibid.*, p. 26.

Spirituality and the Future of Palliative Care

One of the basic objectives of palliative care is to treat the whole person, and thereby address the total needs of the patient. This is not a new concept, and it would be wrong for caregivers in this field to claim that they have discovered a new approach to health care. It may be true that our present health-care system probably puts greater emphasis on meeting the physical needs, but it is also true that expertise in other disciplines is available for patients. In this sense we already practise a multidisciplinary approach to health care, but this does not necessarily mean that we are effectively treating the whole person.

The two words, which are commonly used to describe this approach to health care, are *multidisciplinary* and *interdisciplinary*. We already enjoy a multidisciplinary service, but we have not developed an adequate interdisciplinary service. The latter approach recognizes the need for each discipline to work and communicate with each other. A multidisciplinary approach can easily divide the patient into parts and treat them separately. But an interdisciplinary approach recognizes the interrelationship of the various aspects of a person, and endeavours to see how each discipline can complement the other in providing total care. But there is more to this than just adopting a new terminology or making adjustments in the system. What is required is a particular attitude or philosophy towards what constitutes human life.

Christian theology has been influenced over the years by a number of different philosophies. As the Christian faith spread into Western Europe it began to assimilate certain thought forms from non-Jewish cultures. Under the influence of Greek philosophy it was thought that the world was divided into two parts — matter and spirit. In the human being this was expressed in terms of body and soul. The two were looked upon as distinct and separate aspects, the body often being associated with evil and the soul with good. This was an unfortunate dualism, and really did not reflect the biblical concept of humanity. In the Old Testament the word for body and man was the same. It was possible to use the word *body* with the meaning of self, person, personality, or the whole person. In the story of creation God breathed on the body and it became a living being. There is no evidence of there being a distinction between body and soul.

The way we treat patients within the health care system today largely reflects a dualistic philosophy. It is assumed that the body can be treated separately from the spirit, and that the one has little or no influence upon the other. This does not imply that health-care professionals have no regard for the spiritual needs of the patients, it is just that there is a prevailing attitude that the body and the spirit can be treated separately.

What is needed within the health-care system is an attitude which takes note of the interrelationship between the physical and the spiritual. Some people shy away from the term *holistic medicine,* and yet it describes an approach to health care that recognizes how one aspect of human life can affect another.

Melzack, Wall, and Twycross (as indicated earlier) have pointed out that effective psychological interventions can promote the physical well-being of patients. It would be interesting to consider whether the same tools could be used to measure the results of effective spiritual interventions. Some might argue that the measuring tools used in the medical disciplines are not necessarily appropriate in the field of spirituality. In order to arrive at a reliable statistical analysis it would be necessary to conduct a comparative study within a controlled framework. This would require depriving one group of patients from spiritual intervention. To use this kind of scientific methodology and deliberately deprive a person of spiritual care may be morally reprehensible. And so it may be necessary to devise some other kind of tool to produce credible results. Further study is needed in this field.

Another related issue, which is very contemporary in nature, is the request from ministries of health and various health-care services to develop a quality assurance programme for pastoral care. This raises the question as to whether one can reliably quantify the effectiveness of such work. Some people might simply respond, "How can you measure God?" While I would agree that it may be inappropriate to use the same method of evaluation for pastoral care as that used for medical procedures, it is very important that pastoral caregivers do not argue some kind of divine dispensation as an excuse for avoiding accountability.

It may be possible to develop an evaluation tool whereby certain categories of spiritual needs are identified and a record made of how specific pastoral interventions have met those needs. One such programme is being developed at the Royal Marsden Hospital in London, England, under the direction of the Rev. Rod Cosh. Such categories as the need to love and be loved, the need for hope and creativity, the need for meaning and purpose have been suggested as measuring guides for evaluating the effectiveness of specific methods of pastoral care. But whatever tool or programme is used, it is imperative that something be devised in the near future before an entirely inappropriate programme is imposed on pastoral caregivers.

Before spirituality is accepted as a respectable and useful component in palliative care, it will be necessary to incorporate within the curricula of both medical and theological institutions an educational programme which recognizes the contribution each discipline can make towards the total care of the patient. But this must be done at a very early stage in the educational process, certainly before caregivers become so engrossed in their own specialty that they lose sight of, or become indifferent to, the interrelatedness of different disciplines. If such educational progammes were developed, it might lessen the need for palliative-care units or additional palliative-care personnel within our health-care system.

Another area of concern which needs to be addressed in the future, and it is related to the need for a more effective interdisciplinary approach to health care, is the way in which rituals can be developed that will meet the needs of people facing crisis situations. Kübler-Ross speaks of various emotional states a person may experience in the dying process. How can a spiritual intervention be designed that will help a person cope with these psychological crises? What would be the relevant content of a prayer for someone who had just been diagnosed as having a life-threatening illness? What readings have proven to be effective in helping a person cope with a crisis situation? While recognizing the fact that pastoral caregivers are endeavouring to find appropriate models, there has been very little documentation of those models which have proven to be the most effective. Further research is needed in this area.

The future of spiritual care for the dying will not stand or fall on the number of chaplains in our hospitals. It will continue to meet an important need only when all caregivers come to a clearer understanding of what spirituality involves and what spirituality means to them personally. The thesis of this book is that, even though spiritual care may be a discipline and a speciality in its own right, it is also a kind of care which can become the responsibility of all caregivers. To fulfil this responsibility it is essential that caregivers recognize where they are in their own spiritual journey and what they need to do in order to come closer to achieving the goal of their journey. It is this kind of spiritual evaluation which will enable caregivers to relate more effectively to the dying, and provide a response which will help the dying make this transition in a healthy and positive manner.

"I want people to understand that life is everlasting. Everything that happens in your life has a purpose. There is no one you are close to who ever dies. Every one just goes on to another stage of life that runs parallel to this one. Be at peace with yourself and fulfill your mission, knowing that your stay here is temporary, that you are doing something here to fulfill your spiritual purpose. Tune in more to yourself and understand more within yourself so that you can find your way easier. Don't place so much emphasis on life materially, place more emphasis on it spiritually. Death is not the end, it's the beginning. There is life everlasting, there is no such thing as death. That child, that husband, that wife, that loved one — they are all still very much alive. It's just as if they've moved out. And you may not see them again for many, many years."

Select Bibliography

The footnotes at the end of each chapter contain references for more detailed investigation. The following books have been selected for the reader who wishes to pursue a particular subject, but not for the purposes of exhaustive study. It is also worth mentioning that the Palliative Care Foundation has produced a revised edition of the International Bibliography on Palliative Care and contains a very detailed survey of available literature.

Viktor Frankl, *Man's Search for Meaning* (New York: Pocket Books, 1963).

Viktor Frankl, *The Doctor and the Soul* (New York: Vintage Books, 1973).
These two books explore the human personality in terms of man's spiritual values and the quest for meaning in life. The relationship between spirituality and psychology is discussed at some length.

M. Scott Peck, *The Road Less Travelled* (New York: A Touchstone Book, 1978).
The author provides an integrated analysis of mental growth and spiritual growth, and draws his material from extensive experience as a practising psychiatrist.

Ian Gentiles, ed., *Care for the Dying and the Bereaved* (Toronto: Anglican Book Centre, 1982).
A book which contains both theoretical and practical essays on the care of the dying by Canadian authors who have considerable expertise in this field. It contains many helpful insights for the pastoral caregiver.

Shirley du Boulay, *Cicely Saunders* (London: Hodder and Stoughton, 1984).
This is a biography of the founder of St. Christopher's Hospice in England, who indeed could be called the founder of the modern hospice movement. The story of her life is an excellent introduction for people endeavouring to prepare themselves for more effective care of the dying and their families.

Anne Munley, *The Hospice Alternative* (New York: Basic Books, Inc., 1983).
A study on the practical care of the dying with reference to the spiritual dimensions involved is such care. It is written in an American context but contains insights of universal application.

Victor W. Marshall, *Last Chapters* (Monterey, California: Brooks/Cole Publishing Company, 1980).
This book is written by a Canadian sociologist at the University of Toronto and contains a comprehensive study on the sociology of aging and dying. The author contends that the problems connected with aging and dying are essentially rooted in our need to construct meaning in a continually changing world.

Raymond A. Moody, *Life After Life* (New York: Bantam Books Inc., 1975).
Karlis Osis and Erlendur Haraldsson, *At the Hour of Death* (New York: Avon Books, 1977).
Both books contain accounts of those experiences which occur after a person has been declared clinically dead. The authors claim that their evidence points to a life after death.

Joseph H. Fichter, *Religion and Pain* (New York: Crossroad, 1981).
This book discusses the spiritual dimensions of health care and focuses on hospital and health-care personnel who believe that a religious perspective is essential for a holistic approach to health.

Ronald Melzack and Patrick Wall, *The Challenge of Pain* (Middlesex, England: Penguin Books Ltd., 1982).
This is a technical book on the subject of pain but contains some interesting sections on the psychological control of pain which may have implications on how spiritual interventions can help reduce the level of physical discomfort.

Hans Küng, *Eternal Life?* (New York: Doubleday and Company Inc., 1984).
A book that deals with contemporary attitudes towards life after death and examines the subject as a medical, philosophical, and theological problem.

Harold S. Kushner, *When Bad Things Happen to Good People* (New York: Avon Books, 1981).
This is both a personal account of a family dealing with an inexplicable death and also contains reflections on the problems related to suffering and the existence of an all-powerful and all-loving God.

John Hick, *Evil and the God of Love* (London: The Fontana Library, 1968).
A detailed study of the problem of theodicy which provides a defence of the justice and righteousness of God in the face of the fact of evil.

Bruce D. Rumbold, *Helplessness and Hope: Pastoral Care in Terminal Illness* (London: SCM Press Ltd., 1986).
This book is written for people interested in terminal care, particularly those practising in that area in either a professional or a volunteer capacity. It is not intended simply for religious caring people, although a religious dimension of care is integral to what the book has to say.